REAL SI

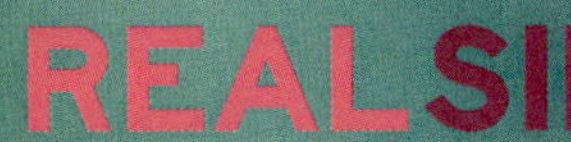

SPECIAL EDITION

Mental Well-Being

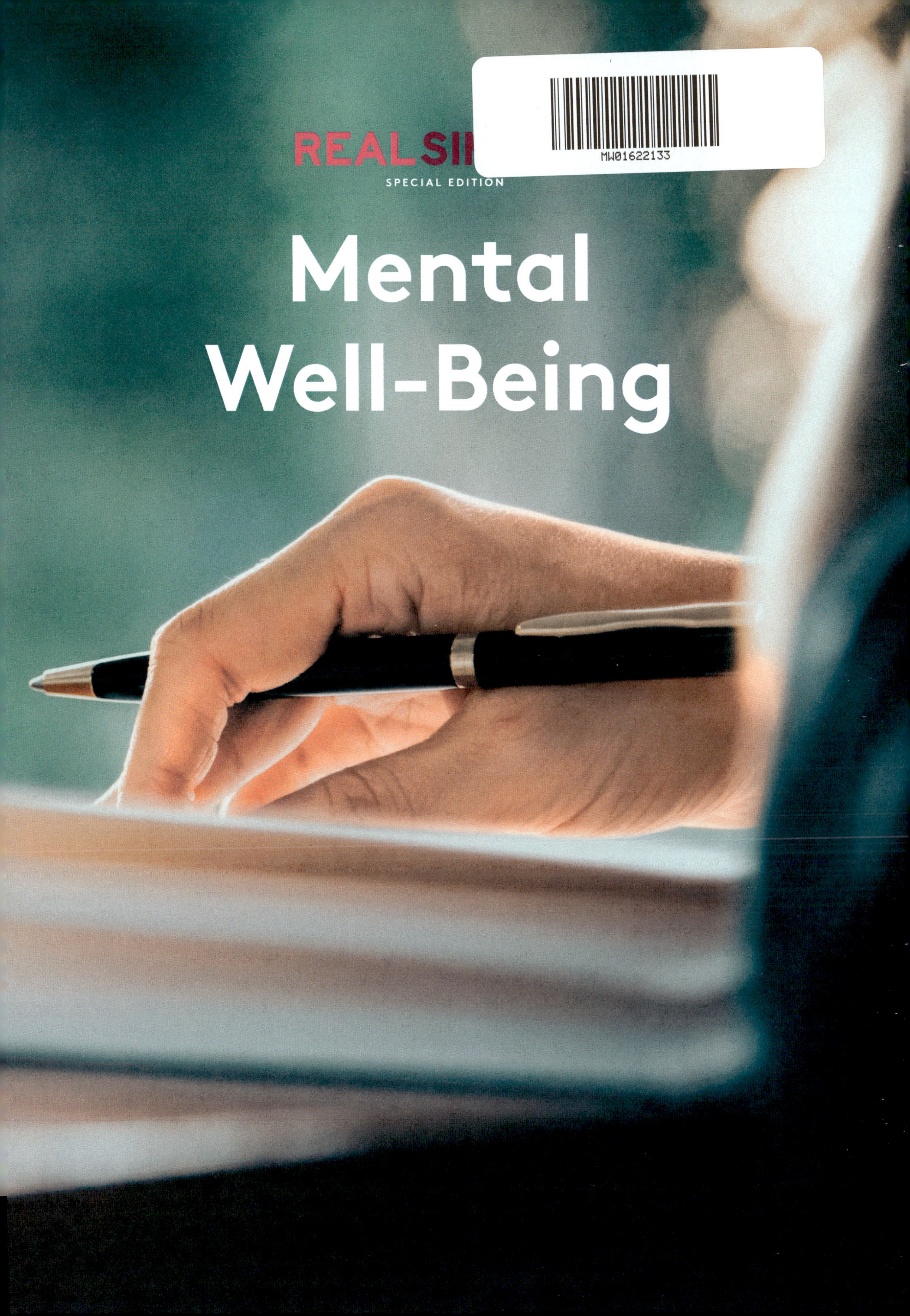

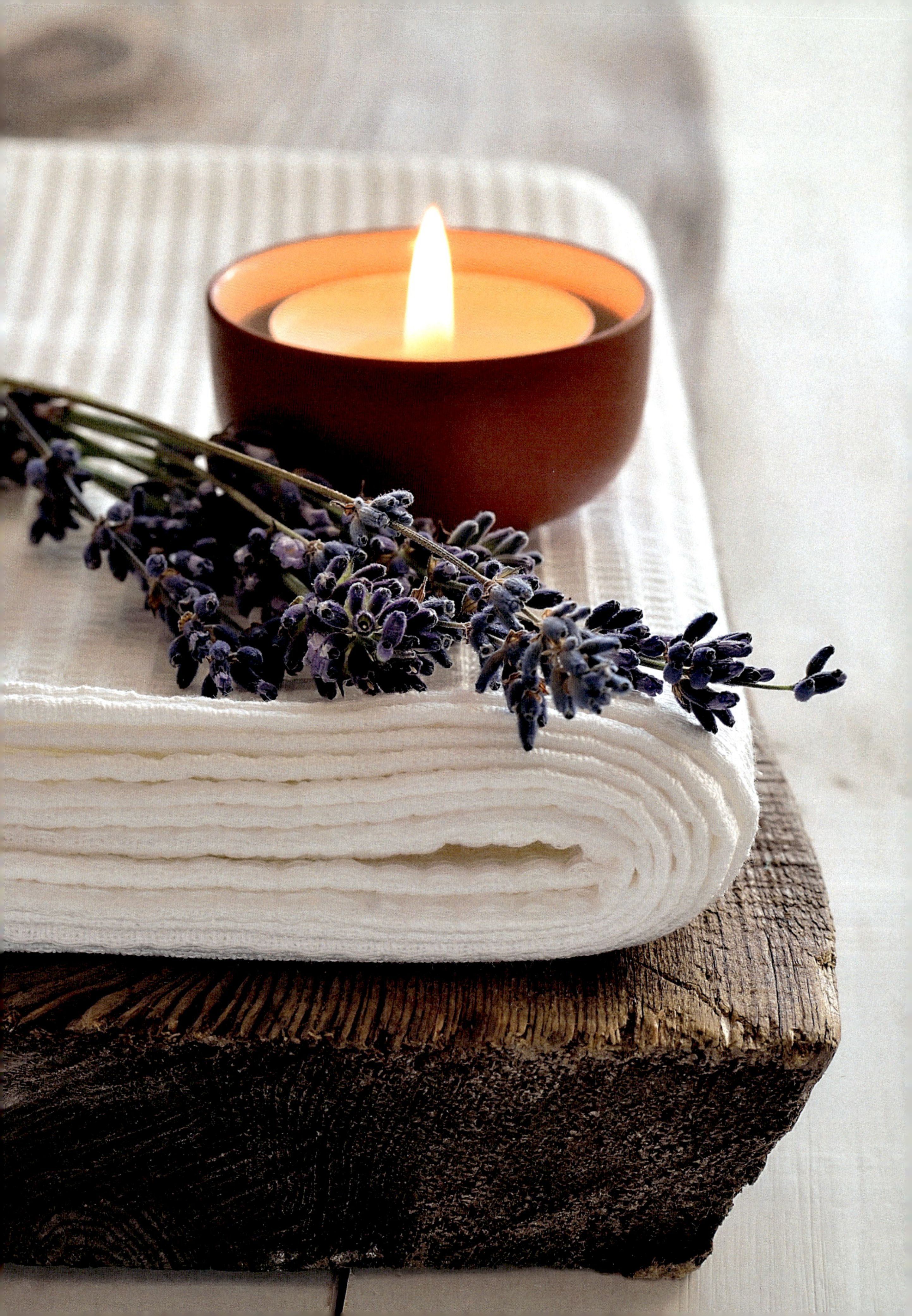

Contents

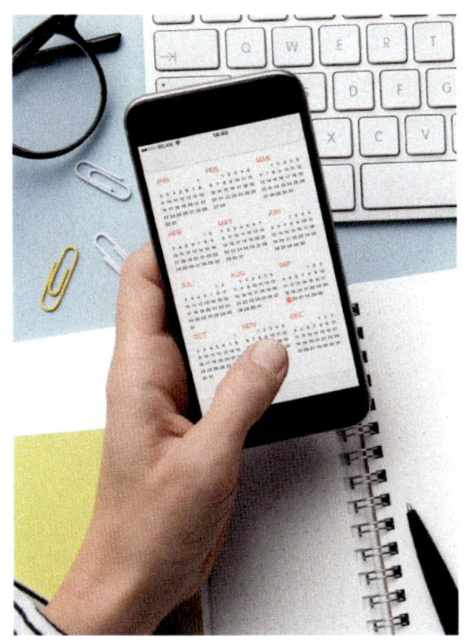

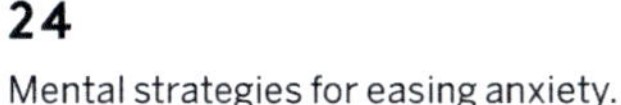

24
Mental strategies for easing anxiety.

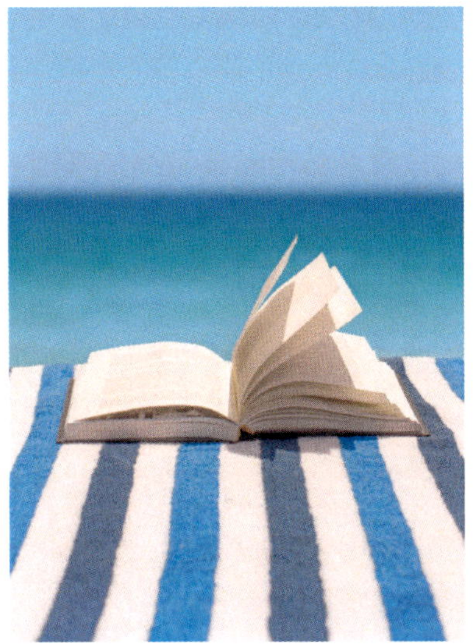

42
TED Talk tips to feel calm and inspired.

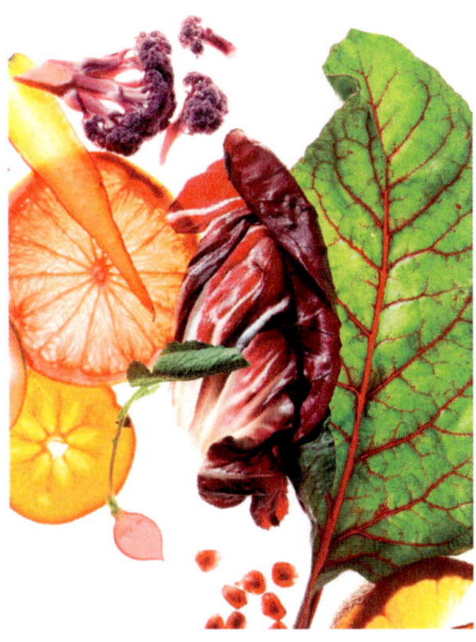

76
What and when to eat to boost your mood.

INTRODUCTION

DON'T FORGET ABOUT YOU

NURTURING YOURSELF ISN'T SELFISH—IT'S A CRITICAL PART OF TAKING CARE OF YOUR HEALTH.

By Lisa Lombardi

YOU MAY THINK YOU'RE on top of the wellness thing because you schedule doctors' visits and (mostly) keep up with yoga and spin sessions. But when was the last time you asked yourself, "Hey, how's it going?"

It may sound silly, but doing a self check-in is a seriously valuable form of self-care. "Your emotional health dictates how you feel all the time," says Gail Saltz, MD, an associate professor of psychiatry at the New York Presbyterian Hospital Weill Cornell Medical College, a host of the *Personology* podcast, and the author of *The Power of Different: The Link Between Disorder and Genius*. When we're not aware of what's kicking around in our brains, she explains, difficult feelings can build up in our unconscious and prompt us to do things that work against what we actually want or need. (See: going back to a toxic ex or signing up to run a third PTA committee.) "Self-awareness is powerful and tends to make most people feel much better," says Saltz.

That's better inside and out. "Anxiety and depression impact the brain and cardiovascular system," says Saltz. Addressing worries and low moods early on helps prevent them from triggering health problems.

Self-care doesn't have to mean candles and mantras, we're happy to report. Instead, it's about giving yourself a daily (or every-third-day) dose of what really reboots you, whether that's reading a few lines of poetry, texting your funniest friend, going for a walk or a run (looming deadline be damned!), fiddling at the piano, or holding a plank to remind yourself how strong you are. Even remembering to sip water and eat something leafy counts as self-care.

Self-compassion enables us to take on small challenges–and even cope when things get unimaginably hard.

That was the case with Keisha Blair, who lost her husband when she was 31. "After my husband died suddenly and tragically from a very rare illness, I realized that intentional self-care was needed to be resilient," says Blair, the author of *Holistic Wealth: 32 Life Lessons to Help You Find Purpose, Prosperity and Happiness*. "If we practice being intentional about self-care in normal times, we will be so much more equipped to deal with a crisis."

Yet many women are taught to not think about themselves and to soldier on, Blair adds. "In certain cultures and communities where women are told to 'just be strong' and there's no room for self-care, people often have a hard time coping when there is a tragic situation," she says. "They feel they must act tough by pretending to be OK on the outside—and that's dangerous."

If you feel overwhelmed or are reeling from a major life change, consider talking to a trained therapist (ask your primary-care doctor for a suggestion). "Your brain is your most important organ, but like any organ, it can become unwell, and if unwell, it needs treatment," says Saltz. "There should be no embarrassment in that."

And when life feels topsy-turvy, don't forget to cut yourself some slack. "You don't have to THRIVE to thrive," notes Saltz. "Thriving through tricky times will not feel great, but coping will feel OK enough to get you through and build resilience." And resilience gives us a secure base to live our happiest life. ●

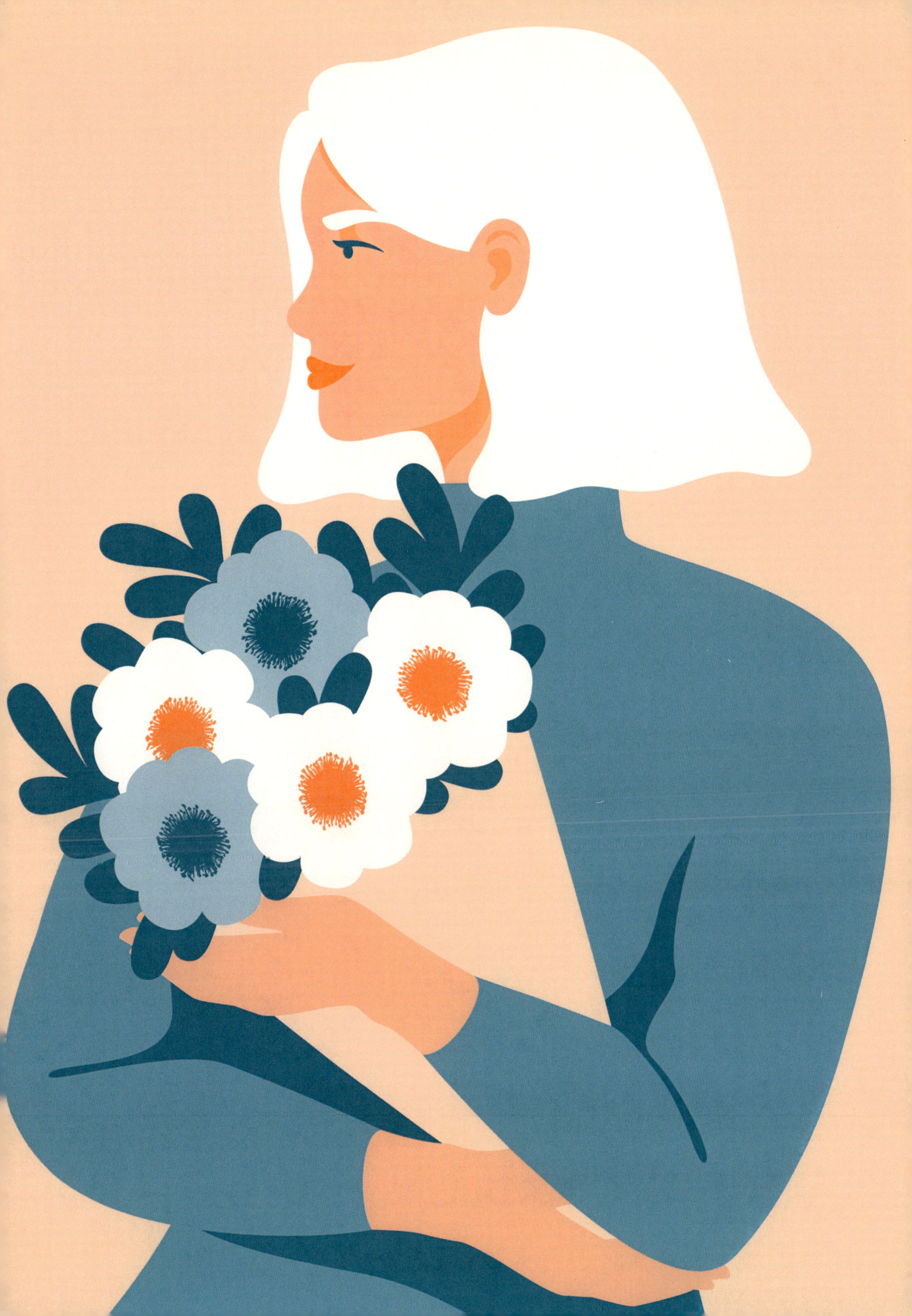

CHAPTER 1

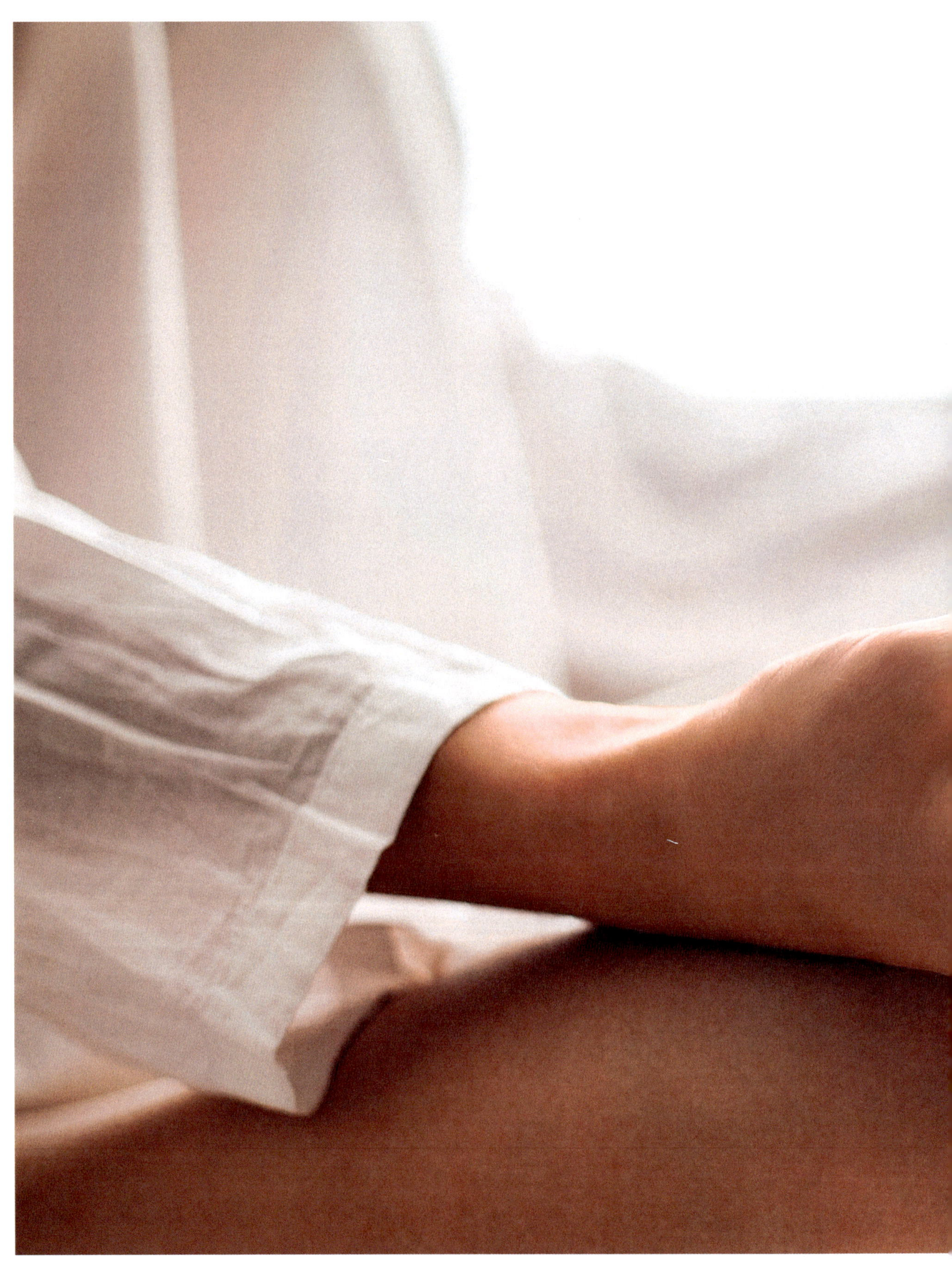

Emotional Wellness

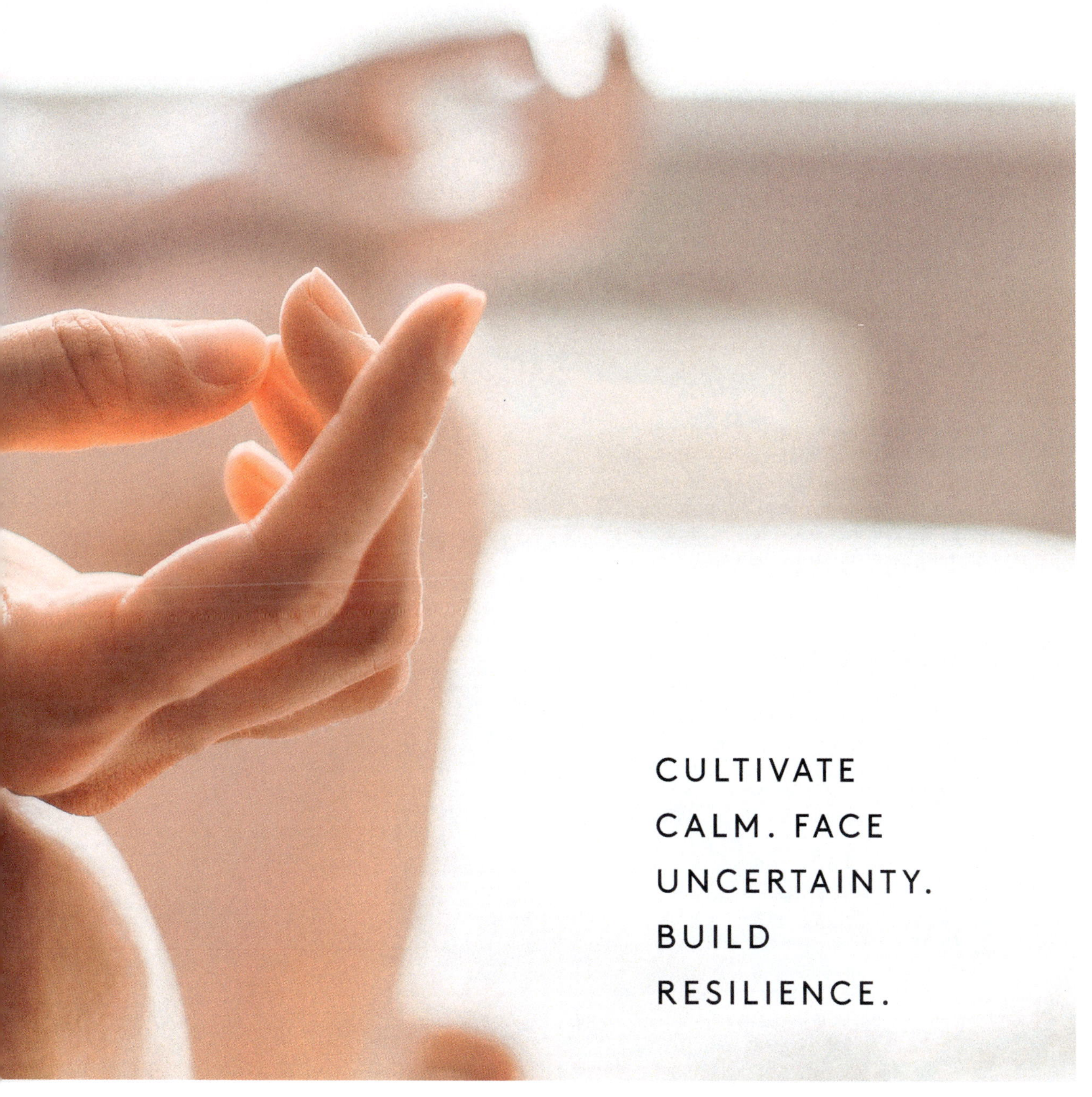

Rewire Your Anxious Brain

WORRIED ABOUT EVERYTHING? AFRAID OF HEIGHTS OR CROWDS? HERE'S THE SCIENCE OF TRAINING YOUR BRAIN TO GET YOU BACK TO A CALM, HAPPY PLACE.

By Ginny Graves

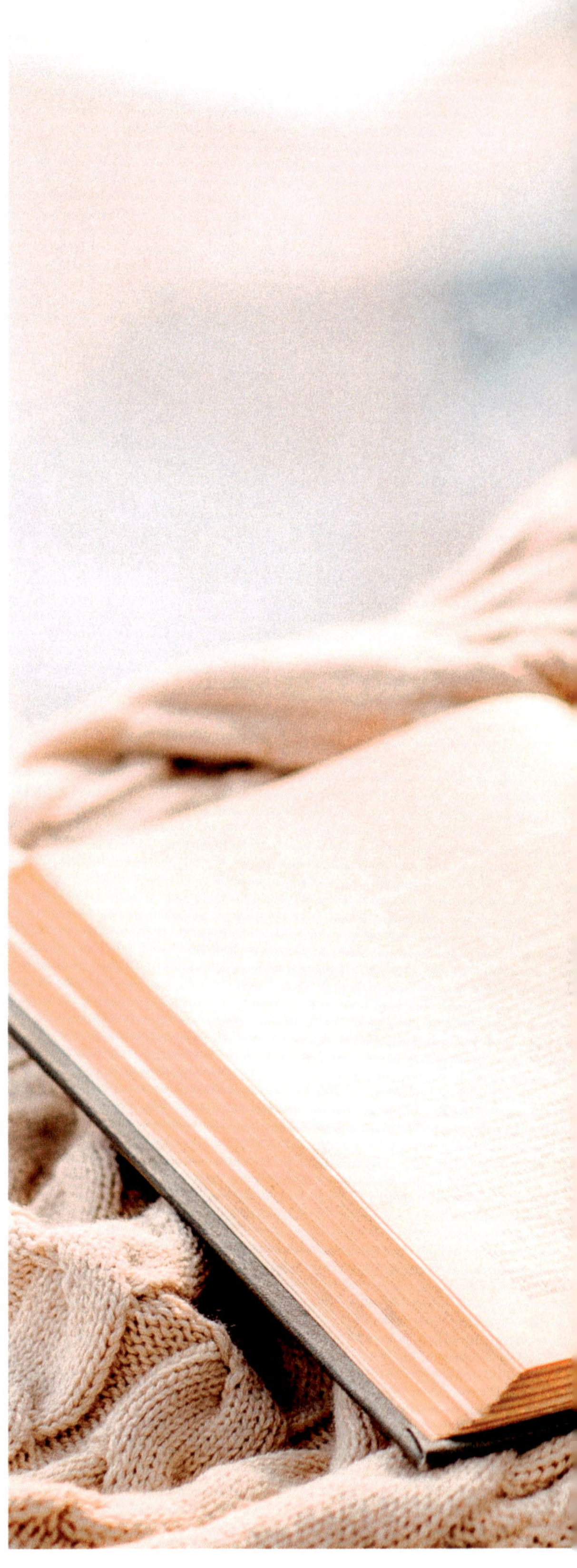

OUR MINDS ARE CAPABLE of magnificent feats of cognition—sending rocket ships into space, inventing drugs to kill deadly pathogens, remembering to buy everything at the grocery store without a list. So why do these same minds also get fixated on fretful thoughts, like worrying that a temporary pay cut will lead to financial ruin or that a partner who is working late is probably having an affair?

Blame evolution. Deep inside your brain lies the limbic system, a roughly 150-million-year-old cluster of structures that developed in the very first mammals to help them recognize and avoid danger. When this system senses a threat, it triggers your body's fight-or-flight response—releasing adrenaline, elevating your heart rate—within a fifth of a second, before your conscious brain is even aware there's a problem. Every time you reflectively dodge an oncoming bus, a snarling dog, or a volatile colleague, this ancient risk-detection network is doing its job.

Trouble is, it doesn't always *analyze*

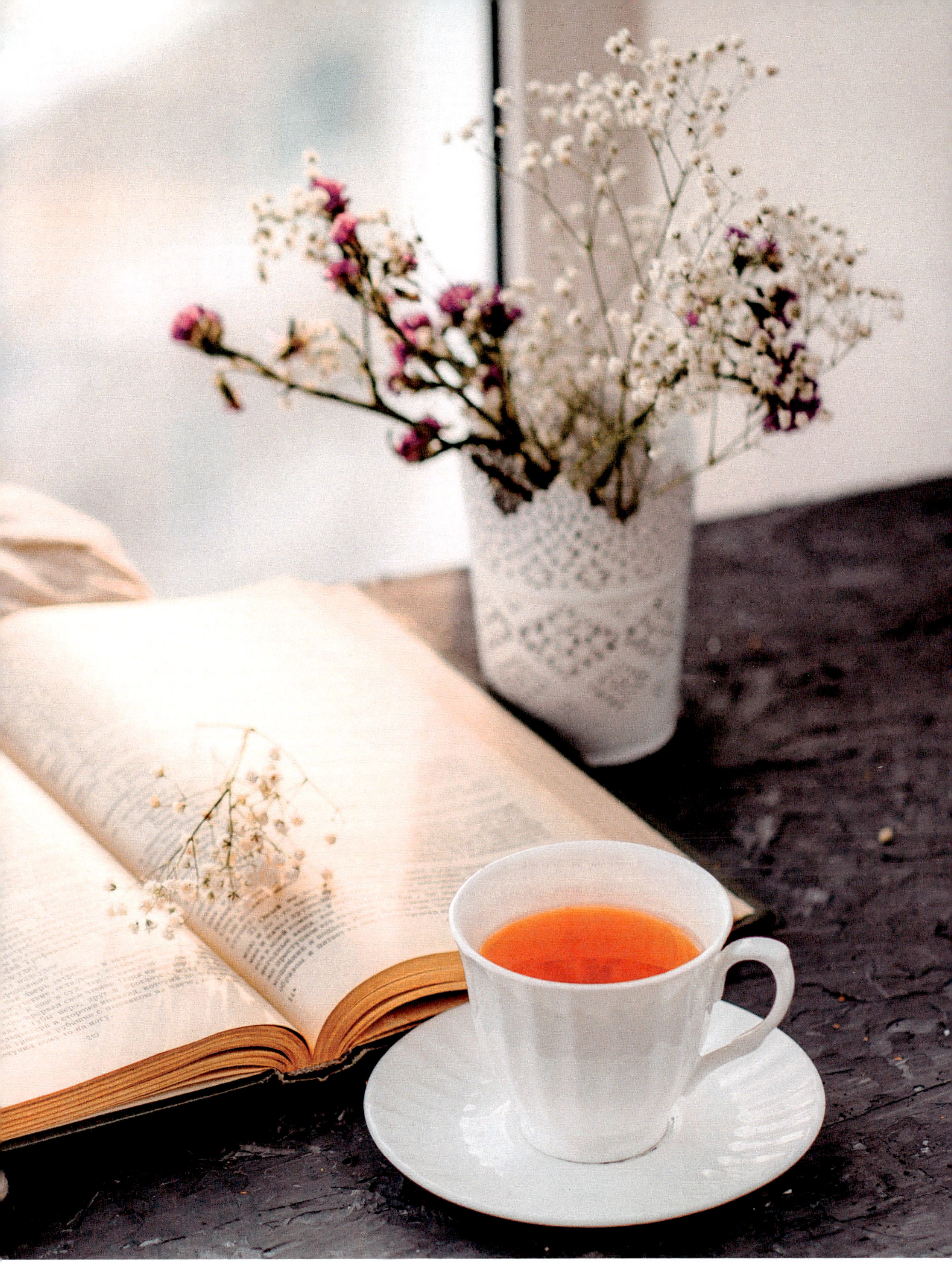

threats. And these days, since four-legged predators are rare, it often interprets mere discomfort or annoyances as danger. "The limbic system can be triggered by things like public speaking or crowded elevators or scowls from neighbors," says Robert Leahy, PhD, a clinical professor of psychology in the department of psychiatry at Weill Cornell Medical College. Those of us who are temperamentally or genetically vulnerable to anxiety (some 40 million people in the U.S.) are more likely to view those benign threats as real and obsessively worry about them.

Happily, our human brains are more sophisticated than early mammals' brains. We have a cerebral cortex, a complex processing area that can do long division, remember to buy toilet paper—and talk our limbic system off the ledge.

Cognitive behavioral therapy (CBT), a skills-based anxiety treatment designed to change problematic patterns of thinking and behavior, offers a variety of techniques to help you reason your way out of a fear spiral, which happens because of how the brain is wired. "Neuroscience has shown that brain networks that fire together wire together, so chronic worry trains your brain to be more anxious," says Evian Gordon, MD, PhD, the chief medical officer at Total Brain, a mental health app.

We can tweak that wiring though. A review of 41 CBT studies published in 2018 found that it was particularly helpful for generalized anxiety disorder, acute stress disorder and obsessive-compulsive disorder. Combined with ingenious physical hacks that rein in your body's amped-up anxiety response, it can provide short- and long-term relief for the chronically anxious.

"My therapist taught me to plunge my face in cold water when I feel a panic attack coming on," says Emily Cahalan, 31, an occupational therapist and long-time anxiety sufferer in Mantua, New Jersey. "The shock of the cold water stops the panic in its tracks and helps me calm down enough to engage in CBT techniques, like questioning the validity of my worried, catastrophizing thoughts."

The idea is to reset the way our brains function. But by learning to replace anxious thought patterns with ones that are less worrisome and more pragmatic, you can strengthen those thought patterns as well. Here are 12 ways to use your analytical primate mind to help your anxious mammal brain calm down.

To gain insight into your anxiety...

Becoming familiar with your anxiety is the first step in taking conscious control of it, says Sarah Gray, PsyD, an instructor of psychology at Harvard Medical School. "You have to be aware of your thoughts before you can change them," she says.

To do that, approach your worry like a scientist. "When you have anxious or worried thoughts, write them down, along with when they cropped up, what triggered them, and what other conditions were present. Were you hungry? Tired? Was it Sunday night and you were stressed out about the coming workweek?" suggests Gray. "Gathering data can help you see patterns. Becoming aware of your anxiety triggers helps you understand why you're anxious and respond more effectively. Maybe you just need a nap." Bonus: Writing about your worries engages your cerebral cortex, which helps you see your fears from a more dispassionate point of view, and according to a study by researchers at Michigan State University, it also makes them less distracting.

Switch on your inner calm

When the hallmark signs of anxiety and intense stress hit—rapid heart rate, sweating, inability to focus—use them as a cue to breathe. "Take six slow breaths a minute, counting to four on each inhale and to six on each exhale, because exhaling triggers the parasympathetic nervous system," suggests Gordon. "It's the single most effective way to put the brakes on the fight-or-flight response."

Ideally, you should breathe like this for three minutes. But if you're in the middle of a busy

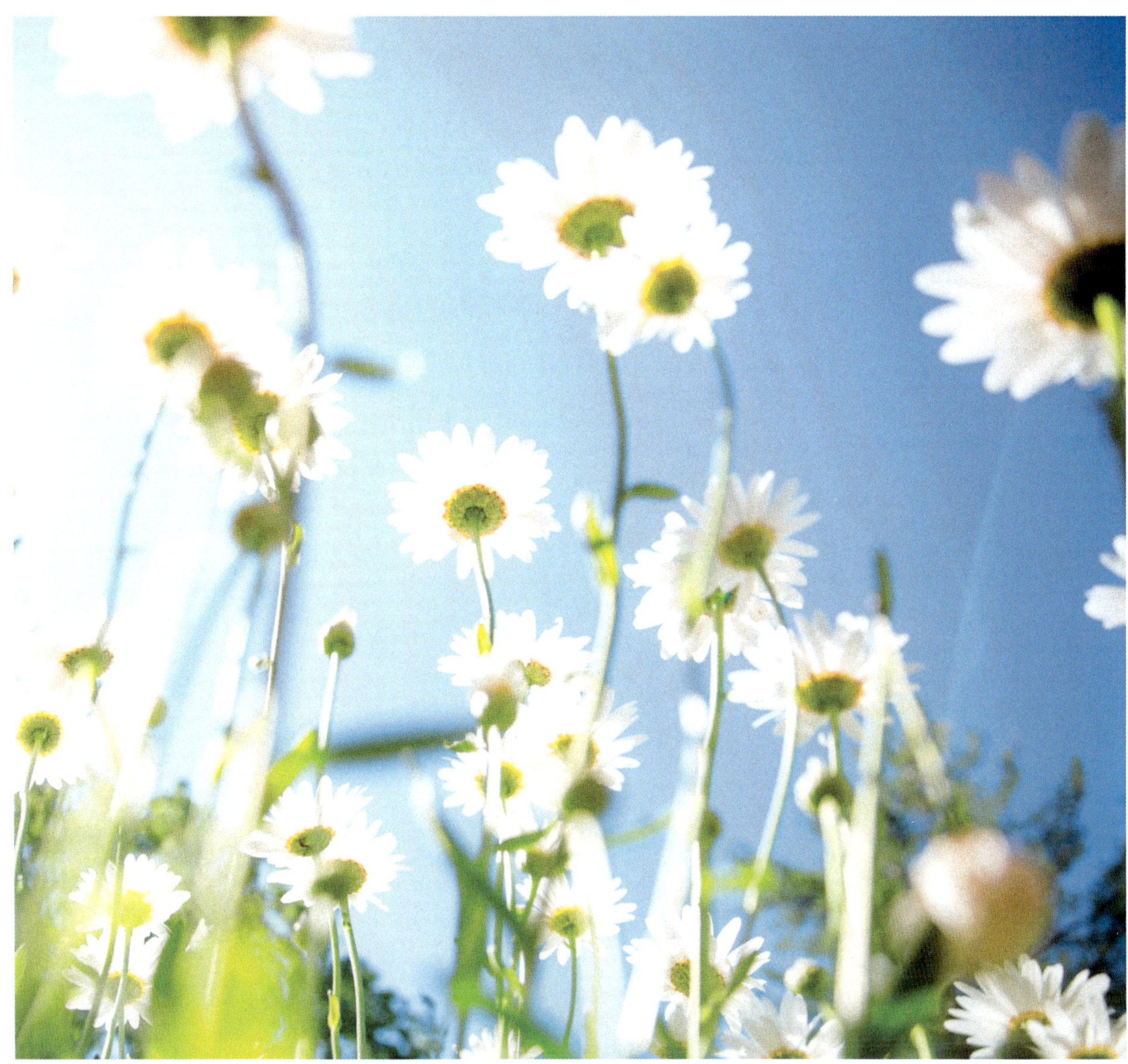

day, even a few 10-second breaths can help you regain your balance, says Gordon.

Get grounded

Cahalan's ice-water strategy is a grounding technique that interrupts the fight-or-flight response by triggering the calming parasympathetic branch of your nervous system. "When I can't immerse my face, I just put cold water on the back of my neck," says Cahalan. Another simple grounding technique: Sit quietly and notice five things you can see, four things you can touch, three things you can hear, two things you can smell, and one thing you can taste. "When you're anxious, your mind is catastrophizing about all the terrible things that are going to happen in the future," says Emily Hu, PhD, a clinical psychologist in Los Angeles. The 5-4-3-2-1 technique brings you back to the present, she says, where, usually, nothing terrible is actually happening.

It's a spin on mindfulness, in which you sit quietly and notice your moment-to-moment thoughts, feelings, and sensations—and mindfulness has been shown to change your brain. "It helps you become aware of your thoughts and sensations—and learn to observe them from a more neutral perspective, so you don't get as caught up in them," says David Carbonell, PhD, a Chicago-based psychotherapist and the author of *Outsmart Your Anxious Brain.* Harvard researchers found that after eight weeks of daily practice, the brains of people new to mindfulness had increased gray matter in areas of the cortex associated with self-awareness and introspection, indicating enhanced function, and their amygdalas, the limbic-system structure that sets off the fight-or-flight response, had shrunk—a reduction that correlated with a drop in stress levels.

Visualize your anxious thought floating away

Your imagination often embellishes and adds to your fears. But you can use this powerful cognitive skill to get rid of them too, says Leahy. "Imagine your scary thought as a balloon on a string that you're struggling to hold on to because the wind is tugging it away," he suggests. "Really picture the scenario. Then let go of the string and watch your worried thought float away in the breeze."

Avoid Google-itis

Odd health symptoms trigger worry because they create uncertainty, which anxious brains dislike. "People Google symptoms because they're seeking certainty, but no website can dispel your fears or provide a definitive diagnosis—so Internet searches only make anxiety worse," says Leahy. What's more, if you combine two terms, like "headache" and "brain tumors," you'll validate that headaches can indeed be a sign of brain tumors, he adds. "If Googling symptoms eased anxiety, people who did it compulsively would be the least anxious—but they're not." Leahy suggests taking a walk, listening to music, or calling a friend when the urge to consult Dr. Google strikes.

Bore yourself with worry

If you're caught in the spin cycle with a single worried thought and can't break free, take away its power by repeating it over and over...and over. "Say it in your mind 200 or 300 times," says Leahy. "When you face your fear, it eventually loses its power to scare you." The technique is especially helpful when you wake up in the middle of the night and start worrying about how tired you'll be the next day. "Just repeat robotically, 'I'll never fall asleep,'" suggests Leahy. "And guess what happens? You doze off."

Be your own (pragmatic) cheerleader

Whether you're stressing about losing a big client or getting your kid into the best school, uncertainty is crazy-making. "I

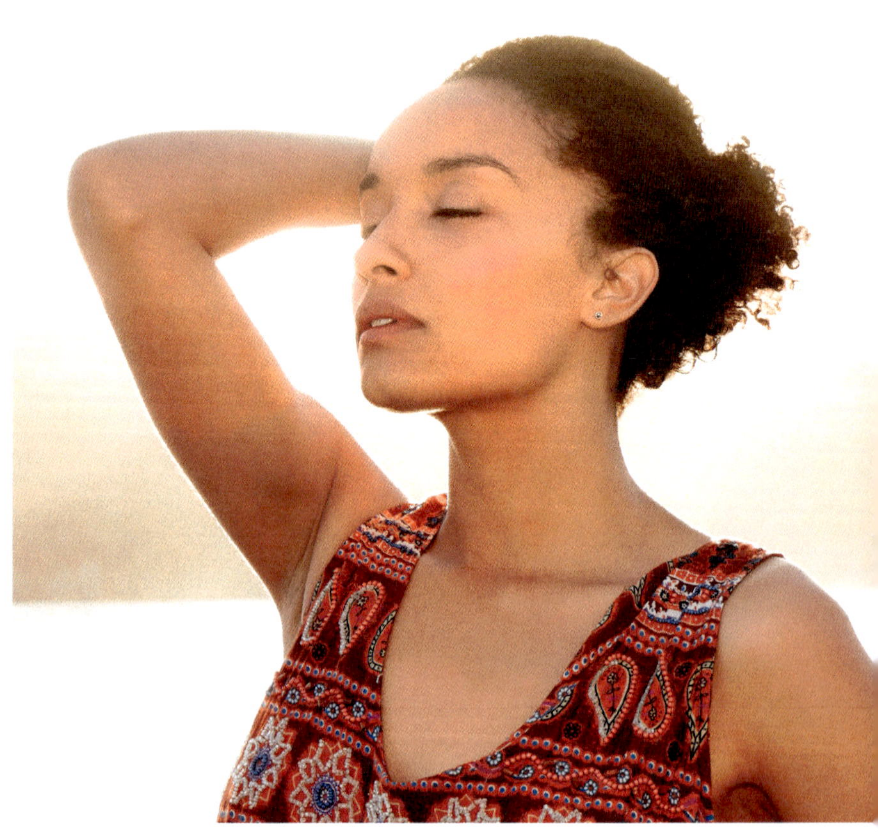

find it helpful to repeat the mantra 'I don't like this, I don't want this and I can handle it.' It acknowledges that life is unpredictable—and that you'll get through it no matter what happens," says Carolyn Daitch, PhD, the author of *The Road to Calm Workbook*. Then replace your fretful thoughts with ones that are rooted in facts: "I have plenty of savings to get through a financial setback, and I could always turn to my friends and family for additional help." Or "My kid is smart and will thrive where he goes to school. And if he doesn't, we can always try another school."

Examine the evidence

"Pretend you're in court and need to provide proof for and against your worried thought," suggests Gray. If you're worried that everyone at your job is judging you, say, identify colleagues who have had your back. Then reframe the worry so it reflects the facts: A couple of coworkers seem judgy, but most are perfectly nice. "This isn't about positive thinking," says Gray. "It's about realistic thinking. Your conscious brain recognizes the truth in rational, measured thoughts."

Call out your inner critic

Anxiety happens when you buy into worrisome thoughts. "But just because you're thinking something doesn't make it true," says Hu. "I've found it helpful to name my inner critic, who feeds me anxiety-provoking thoughts. I call her Yzma, after a movie villain."

Naming your critical inner voice may sound silly, but it is a reminder that thoughts are just thoughts—not necessarily the truth. "I tell myself, 'Yzma is a crackpot. Why should I believe her?'" says Hu. "Externalizing her makes it easier to brush off things she says."

Distinguish between probable and possible

Let's say your teenager is out past curfew. You could think (a) he's probably been in a car accident or (b) he's probably lost track of time. "While the former is possible, the latter is far more probable," says Leahy. "When you're anxious, you're often worrying about things that are unlikely and ignoring the far more likely scenarios. Stepping back and assessing whether your worry is possible or probable can calm you down."

Embrace the gray area

"Lots of people with anxiety struggle with black-or-white thinking—'I always get nervous and embarrass myself when I give presentations,' for instance—which makes the anxiety worse and doesn't reflect reality," says Gray. "Words like 'always' and 'never' are red flags for black-and-white thinking." When you hear yourself using them, challenge the thought. Then come up with a more realistic replacement thought, like "I'm sometimes nervous during presentations, but I usually find a way to power through."

Remind yourself that the feeling will pass

When you're caught in a worried thought or a panic attack, it often feels like the stress is never going to end. "But the truth is, even in extreme situations, anxiety always passes," says Carbonell. "If there's one truth to emotions, it's that they're ephemeral, and that's true of anxiety too." Think about the last time your anxiety was through the roof. Did it feel awful? Probably. Did you worry you might not be able to handle it? Maybe. Did you get through it? You did. In fact, if anxiety is driven in large part by uncertainty, the one thing you can be sure of when you're anxious is that the sensation will ease. So thank your unconscious brain for trying to protect you, and let it know that your conscious mind can take it from here. ●

"When you're anxious, you're often worrying about things that are unlikely and ignoring the far more likely scenarios."

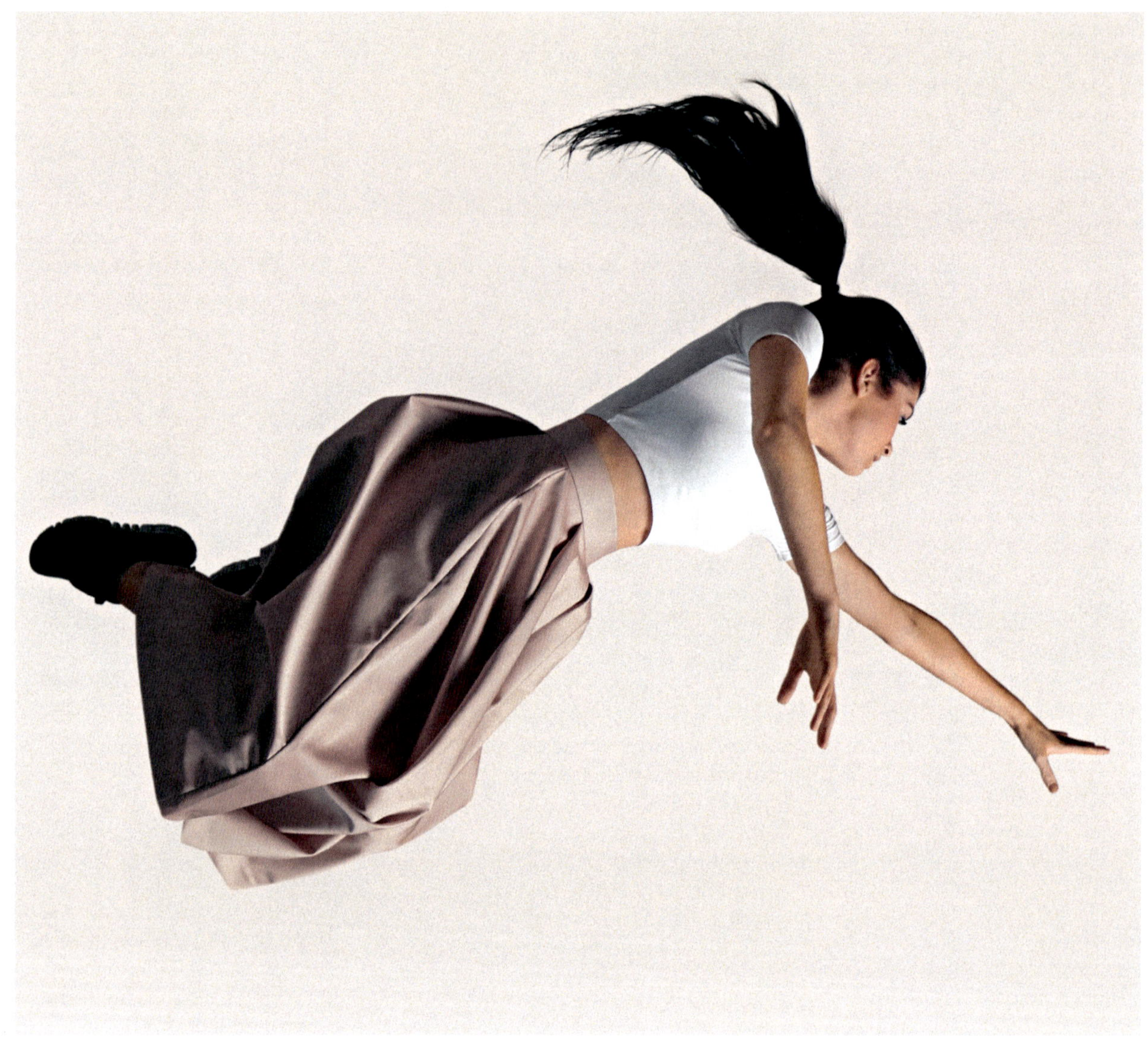

Finding Zen in Uncertainty

SIMPLE WAYS TO COPE—AND TAKE BACK SOME CONTROL—WHEN FACED WITH THE UNKNOWN.

By Maggie Seaver

UNCERTAINTY, lack of control, a shortage of answers—these nebulous unknowns, whether sweeping or mundane, are natural and very normal catalysts for anxiety. Biology is responsible for the unpleasantness we feel in times of uncertainty such as the pandemic, and that is actually for the best.

"When we don't have enough information about the future—when things are uncertain—it makes perfect sense to be anxious," says Amelia Aldao, PhD, a clinical psychologist in New York City and the founder of Together CBT, a clinic specializing in group therapy for anxiety, OCD, stress, and depression. "Anxiety makes us worry about the future so that we can plan for scenarios. It increases our vigilance of our surroundings and engages the fight-or-flight response in case we need to defend ourselves physically," she says.

Why question marks throw us off balance

Uncertainty is anxiety-inducing for everyone, but not everyone is affected on the same level. Research reveals that people with anxiety also tend to have a lower threshold, or tolerance, for coping with uncertainty. Less anxious people, then, may have a higher tolerance for accepting the unknown and managing their reaction to not knowing what comes next.

Think about it. People diagnosed with anxiety or with a tendency to worry might find a social gathering daunting because of all the unanswered questions about the occasion: Who will be there? What will everyone else be wearing (so I can dress appropriately)? How long will the event last? Will I say something awkward? Will the party be fun? How are we going to get home?

On the other hand, someone less prone to nerves isn't bothered much by the ambiguity: Who cares? We'll find out when we get there. I'll just go with the flow.

On the far end of this spectrum are the people who truly relish the unknown. This is the woman who thinks before a party, "I wonder who will be there! I can't wait to see what everyone's wearing—and for them to see what I'm wearing! Who knows where we'll end up or how we'll even get home!" To this type, whatever comes next is thrilling, open-ended, and filled with possibility.

While something minor like a social or work event is enough to trigger alarms for the habitually anxious, some people will feel unsettled only by larger, more existential, or higher-stakes uncertainties—like the death of a loved one or a job layoff.

There's no one correct way of reacting to uncertainty; we are all wired differently. Still, Aldao recommends checking to see if the butterflies you're feeling are in proportion to the foggy situation. "The problem arises when the magnitude of our anxiety response is out of proportion with how uncertain things truly are," says Aldao.

Yes, anxiety is our organic coping mechanism for a lack of control and information. But at a certain point, over-the-top anxiety about something we'd never be able to control or account for is unhelpful and even harmful.

The uncertainty of recent events is powerful enough to set even the least-anxious person on edge. Keep in mind that what you are feeling right now is completely normal. "When things in the world change such that uncertainty increases (like right now), everyone's anxiety levels (regardless of where they were) tend to go up," Aldao says. "For some people this will look like an exacerbation of an existing anxiety disorder, and for others it might mean developing one for the first time."

There is some good news. First, being in a situation that is difficult to predict boosts your brainpower, according to Yale research that was published in the journal *Neuron*. It turns out that muddling through a foggy situation stimulates the brain's prefrontal cortex and prompts the brain to adapt and learn.

Fortunately, there are methods for dealing with nagging feelings of dread. We can't stop hurricanes, bad news, pandemics, or the clock, but it helps to focus on what you can control—yourself. Here are some simple techniques for coping with unknowns, both now and in the future.

1

Tune out unproductive worrying

Not all worrying is created equal. "Productive worries tend to lead to actions that give us more control of our environment, whereas unproductive worries make us feel even more anxious and uncertain (thus leading to a vicious cycle)," Aldao explains.

With this in mind, try to differentiate how much of your fretting is productive (making sure there's enough food in the house) versus unproductive (staying up all night thinking about worst-case scenarios). If there's nothing you can do about it, it's not yours to worry over.

Something to note: Simply tuning out worrisome thoughts is not easy, especially for a very anxious person. That said, the act of taking a moment and recognizing what is and isn't worth the worry is a helpful first step.

2

Be in the now

You can exercise mindfulness when sitting at the kitchen table eating your lunch: Feel the chair under your butt; appreciate the texture of the food as you chew; note the sensation of going from hungry to satisfied. It's not easy, but it's incredibly powerful.

3

Set a routine

Living in unpredictable times upsets everyone's normal schedule in large ways and small. But we can create routines that give us structure and control on a smaller, more individual scale. There is no right or wrong routine, but when you're going through a period when life feels less predictable, establishing little routines may help more than you realize.

"Habits become automatic and give us a sense of predictability and control," says Aldao. "Also because we tend to feel accomplished when we complete a task, they're boosters that can help fight off low moods."

In any moment of uncertainty, the same applies. Maybe you ended a relationship and feel aimless and confused about the future without your ex. Or let's say you moved across the country for a job and don't know a soul. Not knowing how things will pan out is scary, but having some structure in your day and setting small, attainable goals provide powerful pillars that can help you keep going. "In my practice, I've been particularly emphasizing setting up an activity calendar (for work and fun stuff) and sticking to it as much as possible—even if you don't feel like it and would rather crash on the couch," Aldao explains. "This is based on a cognitive behavioral therapy technique called behavioral activation, an evidence-based approach for treating depression and low mood."

4

Focus on what you're grateful for

It's remarkable how taking time to be thankful can transform anxiety. "Finding the silver lining in a new reality is super important," Aldao says. You may not always know the why, how, and when of things to come, but you can reframe your perspective by acknowledging unexpected upsides and being thankful for what you do have. After you go through a downsizing at work, for example, there are pluses: more time with loved ones, no more train commute, and free time to dive into that pile of books.

5

Don't deny what you're feeling

You've heard it before, but it bears repeating: Distracting yourself from the unknown with cocktail after cocktail or late-night cartons of chocolate-chip ice cream is not a healthy way to cope (it's actually a form of avoiding your feelings).

When you're going through a period when life feels less predictable, establishing little routines may help more than you realize.

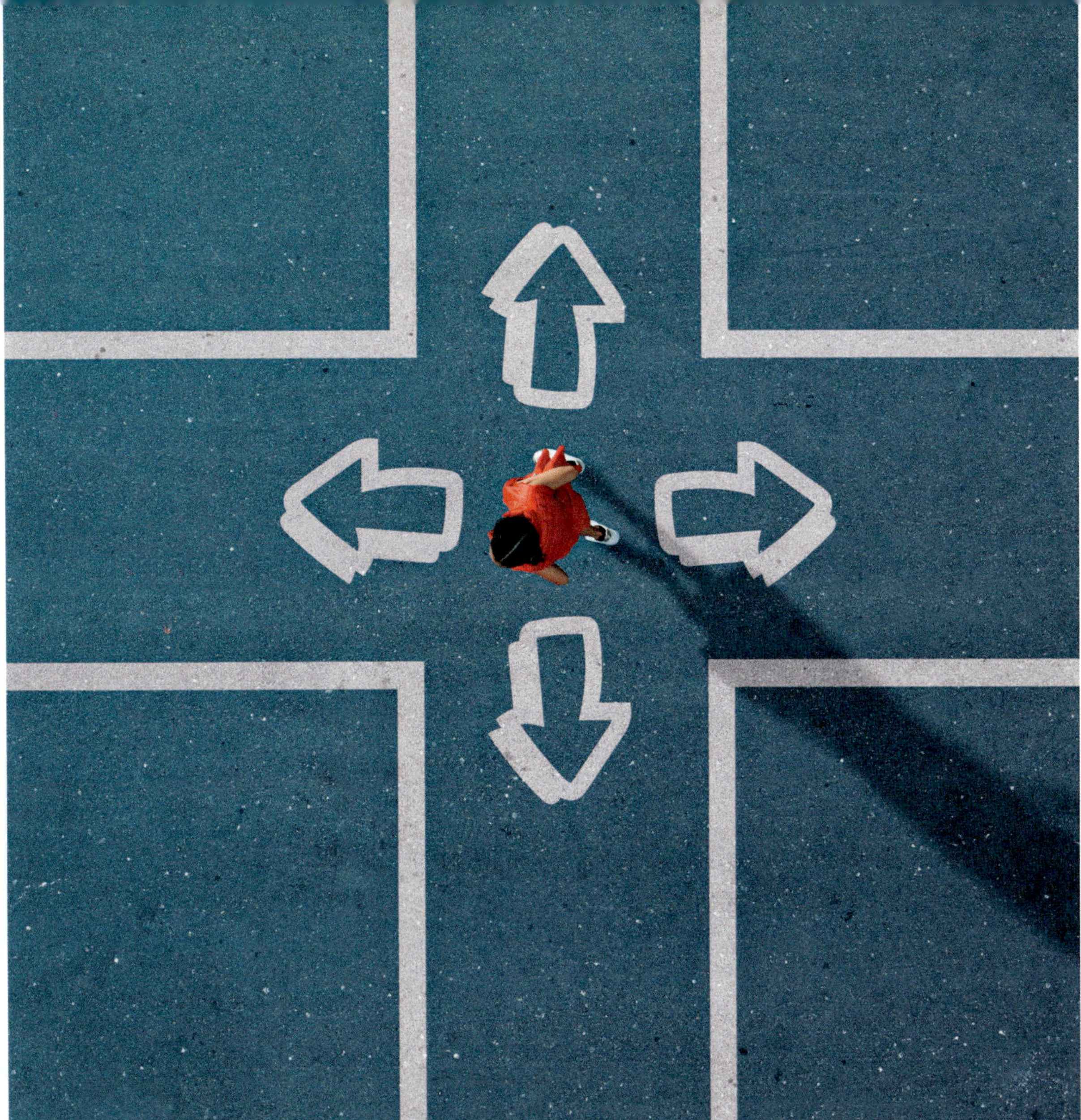

6

Binge-watch something really funny

Laughter may be the ultimate healthy distraction technique out there because it engages your mind and helps you lighten the mood. Laughter also relieves stress in tough times. "Whether it's a TV show, funny tweets, or a group chat with friends, humor is very much about the here and now," Aldao points out. "The more we are in that headspace, the less our minds travel to the future and remind us of how uncertain it is."

7

Accept what you can't control

This move is much easier said than done, admittedly, but accepting the gray area is a giant step toward regaining some peace of mind. Paradoxically, obsessive consumption of information—an attempt to grasp for certainty—can make things feel worse. "Wanting to know and control everything fuels uncertainty," Aldao explains. "Seeking out information is vital, and keeping up with news is important—but constantly refreshing your news and social media feeds only adds to anxiety." And who needs more of that? ●

Bounce Back!

TOUGH TIMES HAPPEN. BUT IF YOU TRAIN YOURSELF TO BE RESILIENT, YOU'LL BE READY FOR ANYTHING.

By Virginia Sole-Smith

"**SOMETIMES IT IS** the artist's task to find out how much music you can still make with what you have left," wrote Itzhak Perlman, the violinist who became a virtuoso despite contracting polio at age 4 and relying on crutches or a wheelchair for most of his life. Most of us don't play concertos. But at one point or another, we'll all be knocked down by life—a sick child, a lost job, a troubled marriage—and have to resume the everyday business of living with joy and purpose. How well you do that depends on your level of resilience, a.k.a. your "ability to bounce back," says psychiatrist Dennis Charney, MD, the dean of the Icahn School of Medicine at Mount Sinai in New York City, who has spent decades researching how people do just that. Charney began his career studying people with post-traumatic stress disorder (PTSD). "It occurred to us that we could learn more from people who had the same kind of trauma as PTSD patients but either never developed the condition

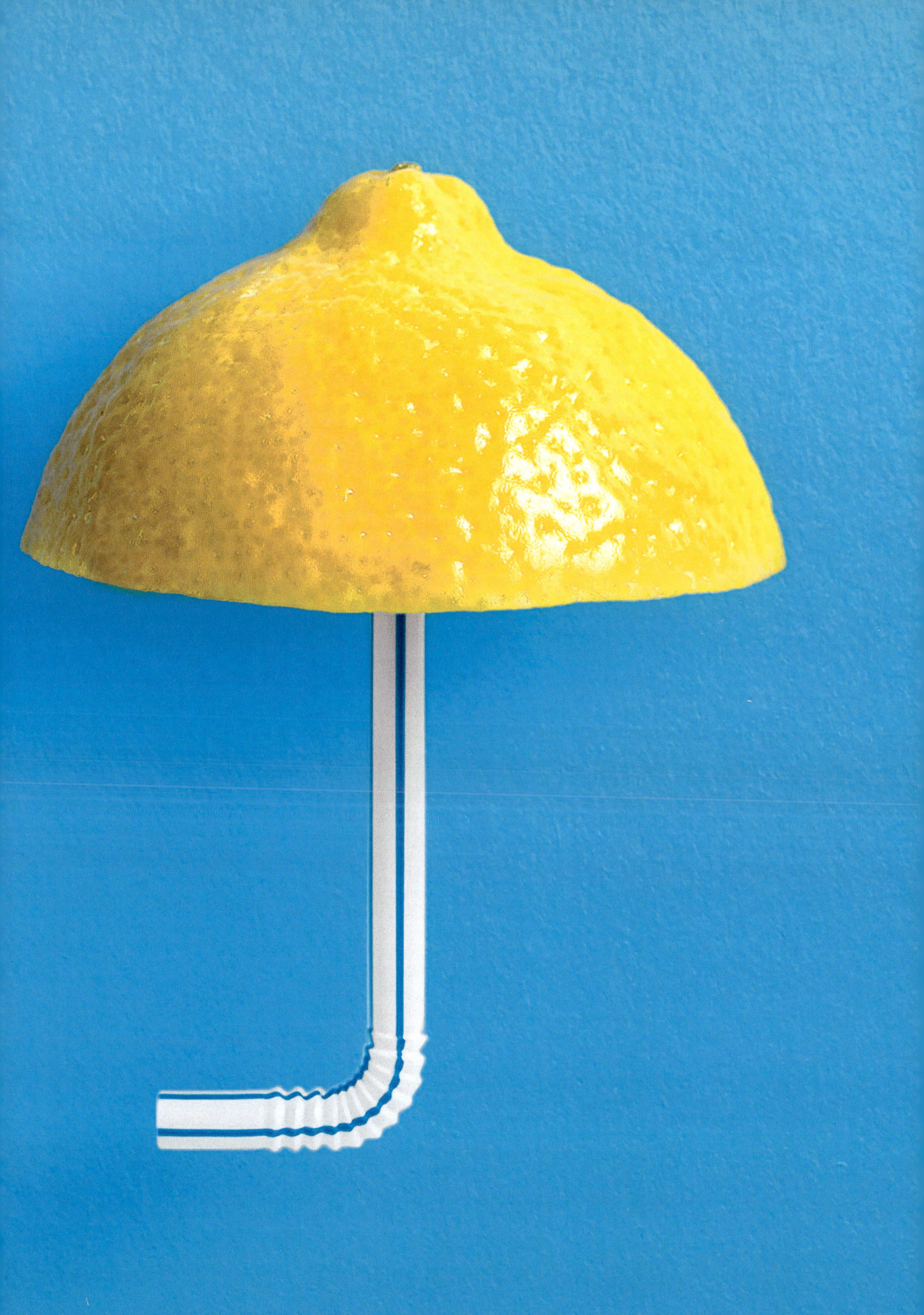

or managed to overcome it," he says.

Charney and his team learned that resilient people are less likely to be diagnosed with mental health struggles like PTSD, depression, and anxiety, which may not come as a surprise. But increasingly, research is showing that the ability to thrive despite difficult circumstances can speed recovery from injury and surgery, reduce pain, and improve health outcomes for a wide variety of conditions. Optimists are less likely to suffer from heart attacks and tend to recover better from coronary-artery bypasses. And people who can speak positively about mild stressors are less likely to need a doctor, according to a research review published in 2004 in the *Journal of Personality*. A 2008 study in *Annals of Behavioral Medicine* found that osteoarthritis patients who are especially resilient experience less pain than others with the condition.

Well, that's great for them, you might be thinking—because a common misconception about resilience is that either you have it or you don't. But it's a skill you can learn and cultivate. "You can move the needle on this," says Charney. Here's how.

Let yourself feel sad

If you've ever reacted to some really bad news by collapsing in tears or getting mad at your spouse, you might think those were not the coping skills of a particularly resilient person. Actually, they are, says Angela Duckworth, PhD, a professor of psychology at the University of Pennsylvania, a founder of Character Lab, a nonprofit dedicated to helping children thrive, and the author of *Grit: The Power of Passion and Perseverance*, for which she interviewed dozens of CEOs, athletes, spelling-bee champions, and other highly resilient people. "They were all very quick to share stories about their moments of weakness," she says. "And I'm not talking about that time you got a B+ on a test. I'm talking about that time you tried to kill yourself, or the years you spent battling an eating disorder. Resilient people are not perfect, and they don't always know what the hell they're doing.

"In fact, scientists have found that when animals encounter stressful circumstances, one of the first things their brains do is activate a 'hopelessness circuit.'" In humans, this can manifest as intense feelings of grief or anger and, sometimes, a profound need to binge-watch Netflix in our pajamas. "We know there's a period of time when you almost inevitably have to feel despondent," explains Duckworth. "There's a neurobiological reason why that lasts for a few days—because it's only after those feelings clear out that hope can kick in." That flood of negative feelings may be your brain's way of grappling with a tough reality: Facing your problems is a key step toward acceptance. "To understand hope, you have to also understand hopelessness," notes Duckworth.

Of course, if hope doesn't kick in, such behaviors can be a sign of depression, so talk to your doctor if more than two weeks go by and you're still struggling. Warns Charney: "If you can't get up and go to work in the morning or you find yourself withdrawing from family and friends, these are warning signs that should not be ignored." Otherwise, let yourself wallow a bit when you need to—and know that your brain is laying important groundwork for a more resilient frame of mind.

Control what you can

Duckworth likes to point to a famous experiment performed by University of Pennsylvania psychology doctoral students in 1967 in which dogs were given mild electric shocks to their back paws. Half the dogs could make the shocks stop by pushing their nose against a panel in their cage; the other half could do nothing. When the same dogs were then subjected to a new round of shocks the next day, the dogs that had control over the previous day's shocks quickly learned they could jump over a low wall to safety. But two-thirds of the dogs that hadn't been able to control anything just lay down and whimpered until the shocks

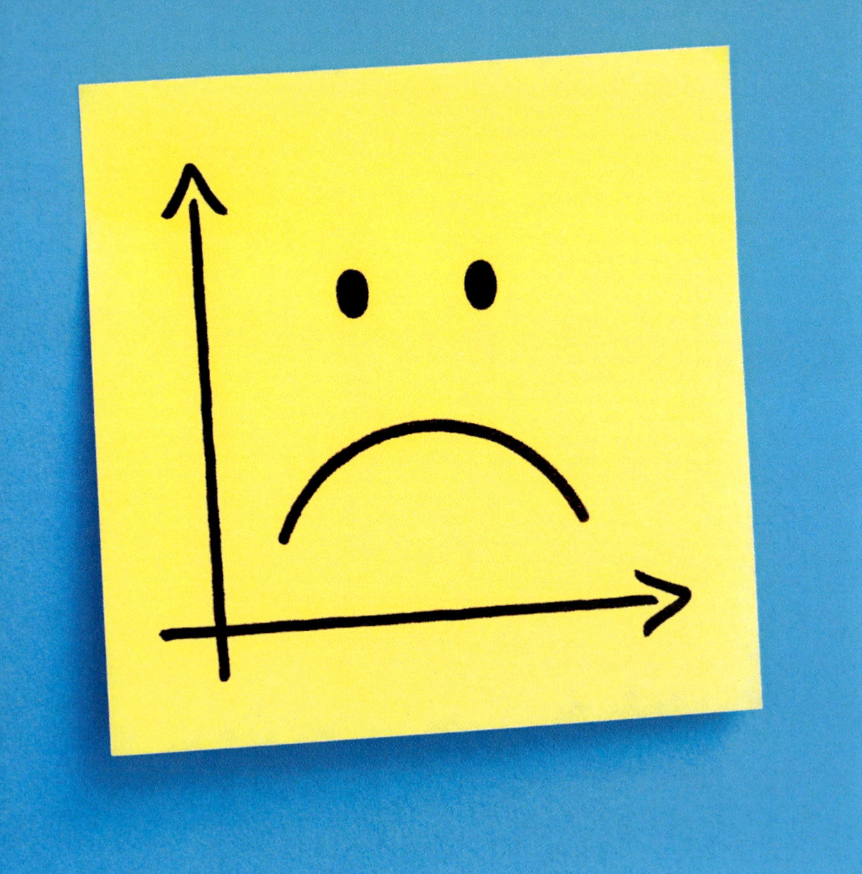

"If you stay focused on what you can control, you avoid becoming paralyzed by the spiral of blame."

were over. "This experiment proved that it isn't suffering that leads to chronic hopelessness," says Duckworth. "It's suffering that you think you can't control."

Of course, we often can't control the outcome of a job interview, surgery, or other stressful experience. But when we busy ourselves with a project related to our problem—whether it's preparing talking points for the interview, joining a support group for people undergoing the same procedure, or just cleaning the house so as not to live in chaos while life falls apart—we're building resilience. "These are all ways of empowering yourself, of saying, 'What can I do?'" notes Robert Brooks, PhD, a psychologist at Harvard Medical School and the author of *The Power of Resilience*. "If you stay focused on what you can control, you avoid becoming paralyzed by the spiral of blame and by asking, 'Why me?' We have far more control than we realize over our attitude and response to these situations."

But know when to be flexible

"People often ask me, 'Is there such a thing as too much resilience? What if you just keep trying or hoping for something that is never going to happen?'" says Duckworth. Her research suggests that most of us are more likely to give up too soon than hang on to false hope for too long. But she also underscores that good judgment is a critical component of grit. "It's not resilience if you're just trying the same thing over and over and expecting change," she explains. "Trying hard isn't enough; being resilient means you're also willing to try differently." This entails developing your problem-solving skills, says Brooks. If you're struggling to land a job in a new field, for example, don't just keep blindly sending out résumés. Instead, sit down with a mentor who can help you pinpoint what hasn't been working and brainstorm alternative strategies, such as a new way to network or a training program that will add missing skills to your résumé. "Step back, consider different options, pick a course of action, and then assess how well this new strategy works," he advises. "Good problem-solvers think of new solutions and make necessary changes to their approach."

You also need to hone what Charney calls "cognitive flexibility," or the ability to reevaluate a traumatic experience in order to grow and recover. For the book he coauthored, *Resilience: The Science of Mastering Life's Greatest Challenges*, Charney interviewed a family friend who was born with spina bifida. "She accepted the reality of her condition, but she didn't let it limit her view of herself. She learned to swim, and she got

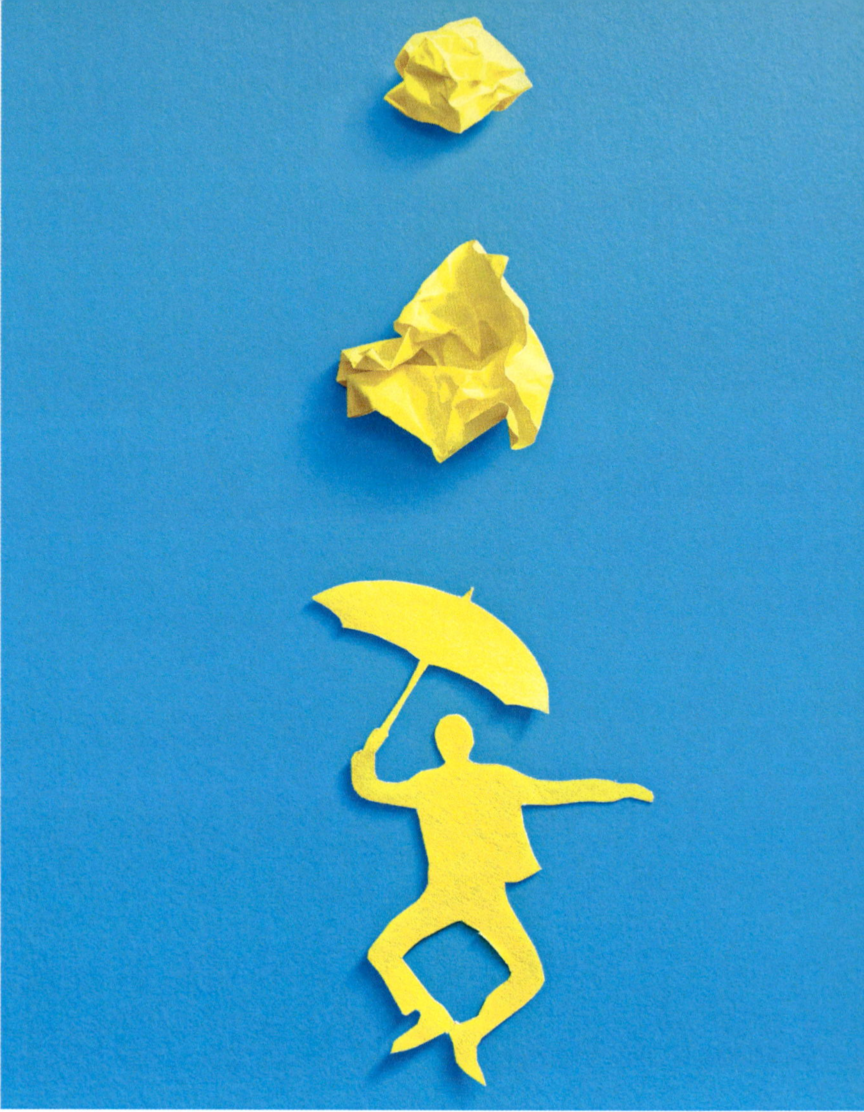

into Yale," he recalls. "Cognitive flexibility doesn't mean you have to find good in a bad thing, because sometimes there is no good. It means you don't let this bad thing define you." For disappointments, like a book proposal that didn't sell, you might be able to find silver linings fairly quickly; perhaps the failed book sparks a better idea. For major catastrophes, such as the death of a loved one, you may need to enlist a therapist to help you find peace.

Find resilient role models

Maybe your role model is your mother, who was the first woman in her family to go to college. Your role models don't need to be people who have dealt with the same challenges you're facing; they just need to have traits or strategies that you can emulate. "The goal is to put together your own road map toward recovery," says Charney. "Imitation is a very powerful way of learning to be resilient."

Be a role model too

"It's important to pay it forward," says Charney—and not just because it's the nice thing to do. Studies show that altruism is key to resilience, and thus good health. People over 55 who volunteered with two or more organizations, for example, had a 44 percent lower chance of dying during a study than nonvolunteers, according to researchers at the University of California at Berkeley.

When Brooks surveyed 1,500 adults about their early educational experiences, he found that a majority considered a time when they had been asked to help out as essential to building self-esteem and motivation. "Decades later, they remembered when a teacher asked them to tutor another student or help pass out the milk," he says. "Helping others makes us feel competent, improves our problem-solving abilities, and gives us a larger sense of purpose. All of that translates to more resilience."

Talk it out

If you have people in your life who believe in your ability to learn and do better—even when you screw up—that will help you view the glass as half full.

This doesn't mean you need your friends to give you constant pep talks. It can be enough just to have people in your life who understand what you're going through. When Charney interviewed former prisoners of war, he learned they had spent hours developing a secret code of taps that allowed them to communicate with one another through the walls of their cells. Women may be especially good at connecting with others facing similar obstacles: "The natural response to stress in women and girls is to reach out, to talk, to share—to feel like, 'OK, I'm not the only one who is failing,'" says Judith V. Jordan, PhD, the director of the Jean Baker Miller Training Institute at Wellesley College in Wellesley, Massachusetts. "Culturally, we're taught that this is a sign of weakness, that you should be able to get it together on your own—but I believe it's resilience in action."

Know that you're already doing it

It's fine to hate the worrisome circumstances you're in, but consider this benefit: By overcoming stress, you become more resilient. "You can't just watch *Chariots of Fire* and be more resilient," says Duckworth. "You have to be in the race yourself, lose, and then see that it's not the end of the world." Going through these kinds of ordeals fires up what psychologists call our neurological hope circuit—the purpose of which is to inhibit our hopelessness circuit and override the neurons that trigger feelings of despair. If your current problem feels overwhelming, remember how you persevered in the past. In Duckworth's interviews with "paragons of grit," she says many of them had a formative experience that inspired them. "When you can say, 'At least this isn't as hard as that was'—that's true grit," says Duckworth. "Be biased toward hope." ●

STRENGTH IN NUMBERS

These inspiring quotes are a reminder of the amazing flexibility of the human spirit. Hang them on your mirror the next time you need to tap into your own inner resilience reserves.

If your heart is broken, make art with the pieces.

—SHANE KOYCZAN, "BLUEPRINT FOR A BREAKTHROUGH," TEDx TALK, 2013

I was set free, because my greatest fear had been realized, and I was still alive, and I still had a daughter whom I adored, and I had an old typewriter and a big idea. And so rock bottom became the solid foundation on which I rebuilt my life.

—J.K. ROWLING, HARVARD UNIVERSITY COMMENCEMENT SPEECH, 2008

The human capacity for burden is like bamboo—far more flexible than you'd ever believe at first glance.

—JODI PICOULT, *MY SISTER'S KEEPER*

Although the world is full of suffering, it is full also of the overcoming of it.

—HELEN KELLER, "OPTIMISM: AN ESSAY"

Yet it seems like the more abuse I get, the more abuse I court—baring myself more extravagantly, professing opinions that I know will draw an onslaught—because, after all, if I've already adjusted my body temperature, why not face the blizzard so that other women don't have to freeze?

—LINDY WEST, *SHRILL: NOTES FROM A LOUD WOMAN*

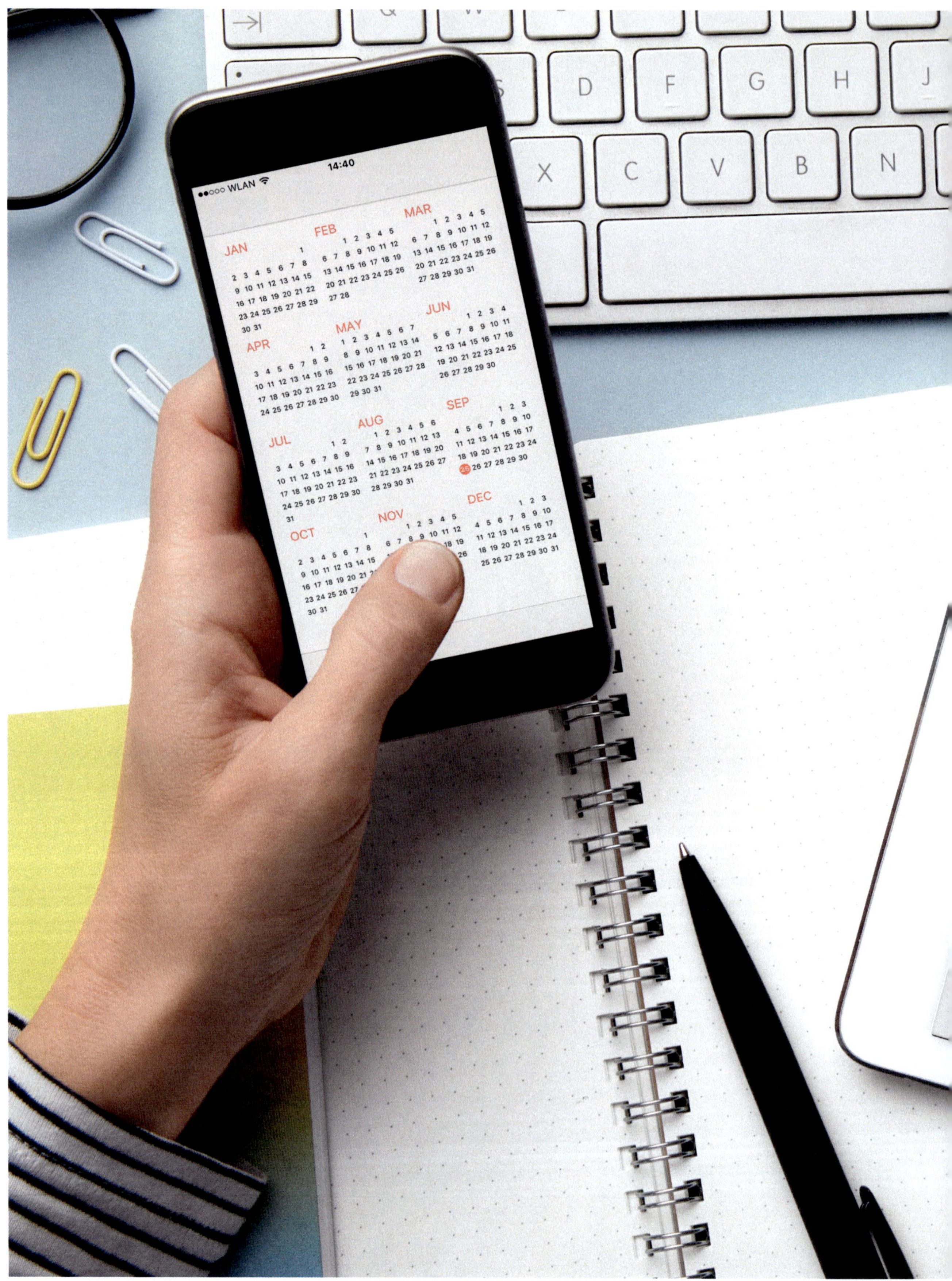
14:40
WLAN
JAN
FEB
MAR
APR
MAY
JUN
JUL
AUG
SEP
OCT
NOV
DEC
D
F
G
H
J
X
C
V
B
N

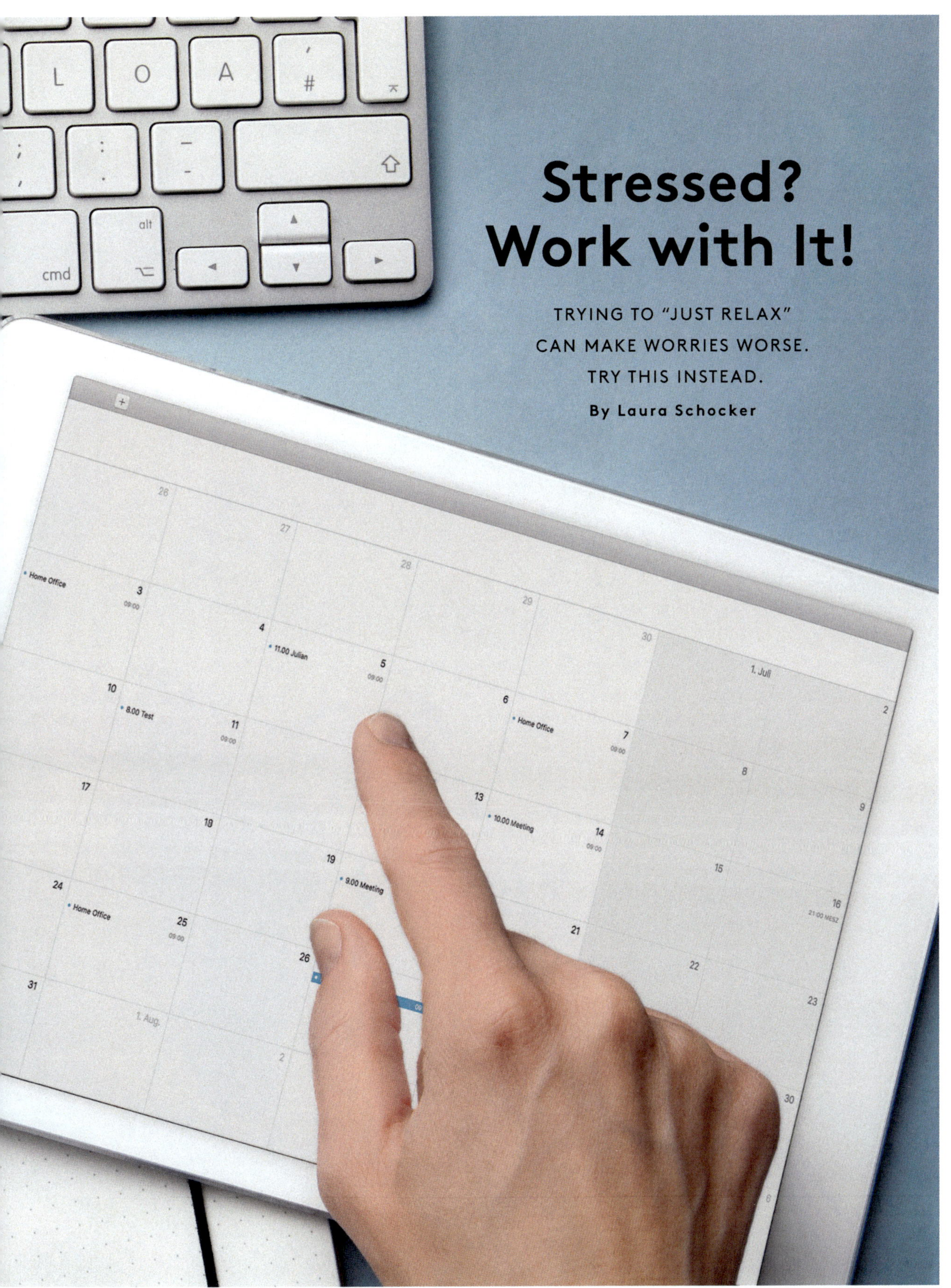

Stressed? Work with It!

TRYING TO "JUST RELAX" CAN MAKE WORRIES WORSE. TRY THIS INSTEAD.

By Laura Schocker

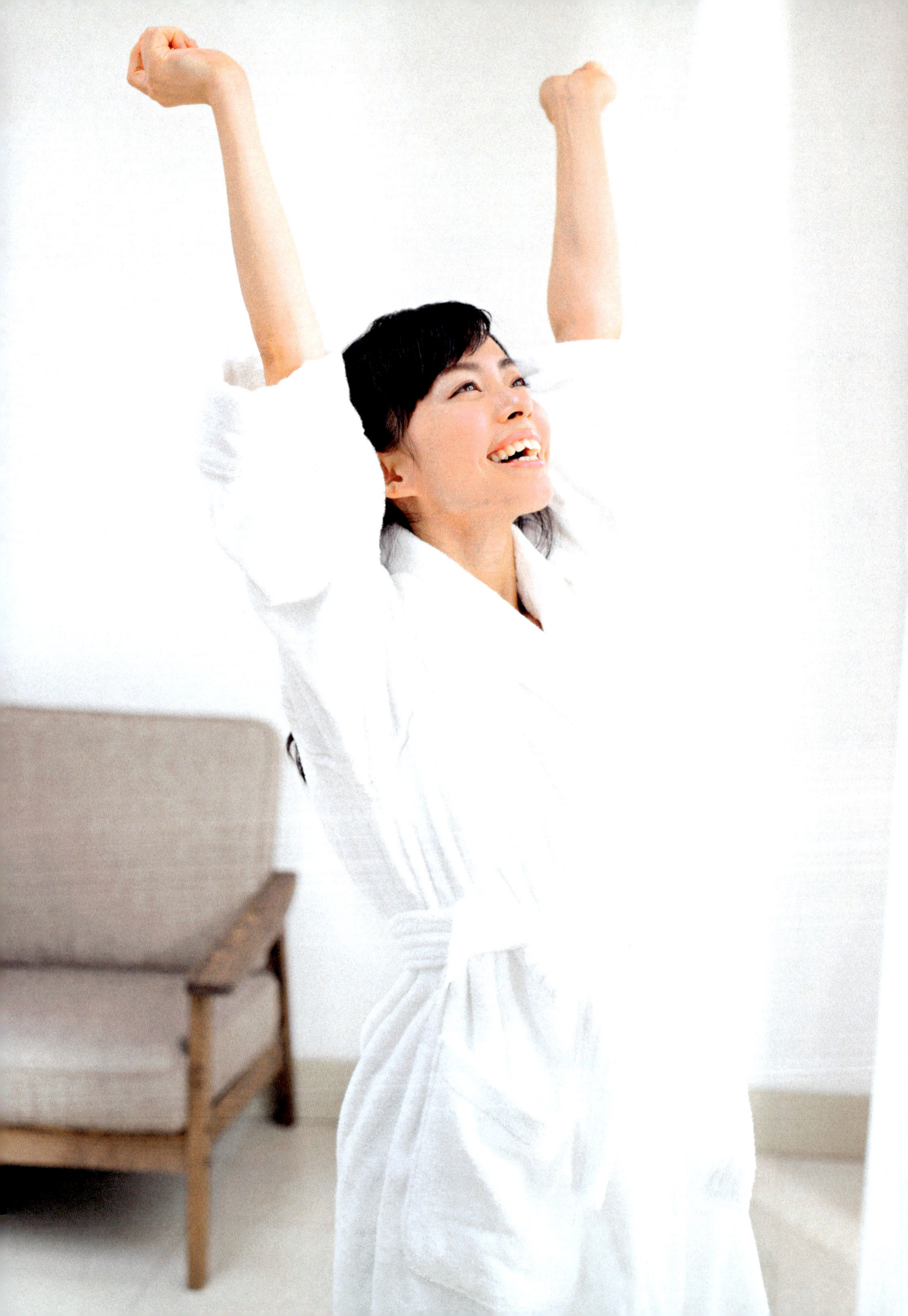

MAYBE YOUR HEART begins pounding and your hands go clammy just before a major presentation. Or you're headed out for a weekend at your always critical in-laws' and your stomach starts churning as soon as you carry your suitcase out the door. The classic advice: "Just relax! Take a deep breath, picture yourself on a beach, chill out." But while you might *like* to cool off, it's really freaking annoying to hear "Relax!" when your nerves are shot, your head is spinning, and you couldn't sleep the night before.

That's because, experts say, trying to force relaxation is like showing up to a black-tie event in athleisure: There's little you can do to switch into the right mode.

"The difficulty with telling yourself to relax when you're feeling anxious is that the bodily symptoms and mental symptoms of relaxation are the opposite of those of stress and anxiety," says Ian Robertson, PhD, T. Boone Pickens Distinguished Research Scientist at the Center for Brain Health at University of Texas, Dallas, and the author of *The Stress Test*.

When you're stressed, your breathing and heart rate speed up, your muscles tense, and your mouth feels like sandpaper. And when you're calm, your breathing and heart rate are slow, your muscles are relaxed, and your mouth feels just fine. No matter how much you may want to calm down, the mental journey from stressed to relaxed takes a lot more time than you probably have before the high-stakes event begins.

So, counterintuitively, relaxing can be really hard work, on top of whatever stressful situation you're already facing down. With lots of practice—regular deep breathing, relaxation exercises, and the like—you might master it, but in the midst of a pre-public-speaking mini breakdown? A few breaths probably won't cut it. It turns out that experts and research say there might be more effective ways to handle day-to-day stress and anxiety (not to be confused with a full-blown anxiety disorder, which goes far beyond temporary stress; the experts all agree that if anxiety is interfering with your life, work, or family, it's time to talk to your doctor). The key, as with any healthy habit, is figuring out which tricks work best for you.

1

Get yourself pumped

Worry and relaxation are diametrically opposed emotions, but there's one positive feeling that's much closer to stress: excitement. After all, you can also get a racing heart or sweaty palms when you're excited. For a study published in the *Journal of Experimental Psychology*, researcher Alison Wood Brooks, PhD, told people they would have to either perform a song, speak in public, or complete a difficult, timed math problem. In each experiment, the participants said some variation of "I am calm," "I am excited," or "I am nervous." The results consistently showed that the ones who stated aloud that they were excited about the challenge performed better across all three categories. "Those feelings of anxiety and excitement have a profound effect on subsequent performance," says Brooks, an O'Brien associate professor at Harvard Business School. "People who said they were excited were better at doing the math, more energetic, more competent, and more persuasive. They even sang better."

This technique is called emotional reappraisal, and it's all about relabeling one emotion as another. One way to practice it is to create calendar invites or leave yourself notes as reminders to get jazzed for an approaching event, suggests Brooks: *Start feeling fired up! Big speech on the 30th.* Or tell yourself a different story about the physical symptoms your body is exhibiting. Before a job interview, for instance, you might think, "My stomach has butterflies because I am so eager to ace this interview" or "My heart is racing because I'm excited for this meeting."

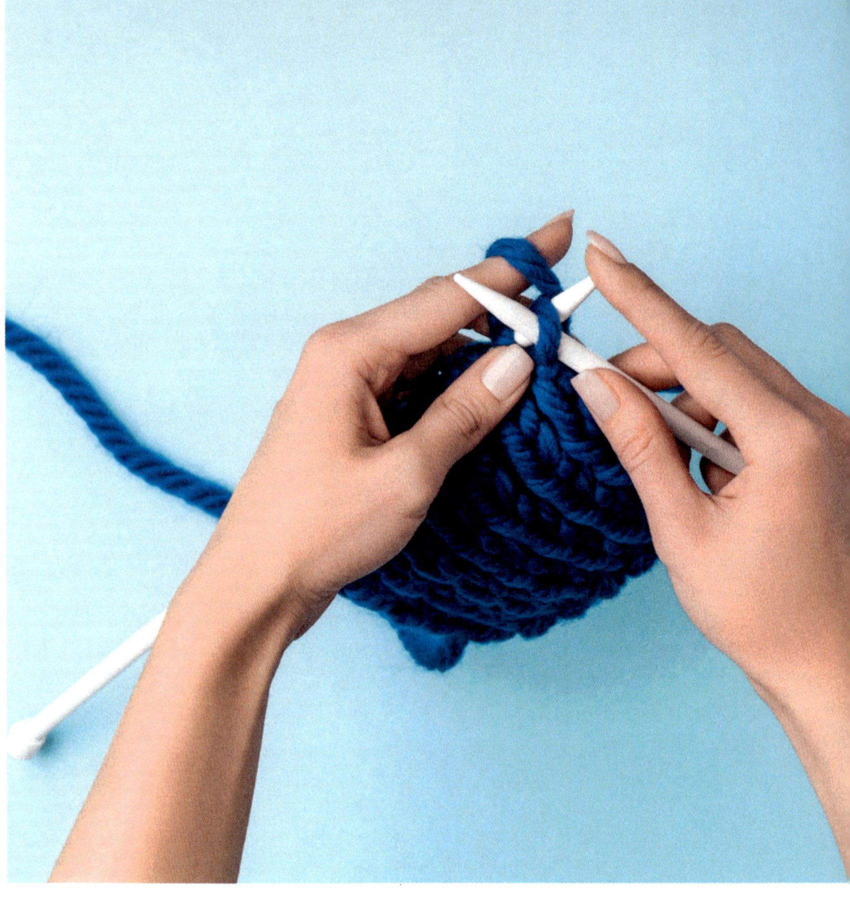

2

Take some action

If there's a looming to-do stressing you out, sometimes buckling down and, well, *doing* something about it is a whole lot more productive than any number of calming techniques could ever be. "Ask yourself, 'Is there a problem here that I can solve? Would solving it lead me to less stress?'" suggests Simon Rego, PsyD, a chief psychologist at Montefiore Medical Center/Albert Einstein College of Medicine in New York City. To get started, break the project down into small pieces. "Chunk it and reduce it until you say, 'That I can do,'" he advises. Say you're so nervous about going to the dentist that you've been putting off making an appointment for two years. Every time you think about it, you get so anxious that you can't deal with it, so you distract yourself until you forget about it. In your list of life stressors, it's The Dentist (*dun dun dunnn...*), and it feels untouchable. Break it down until it feels doable: (1) Ask three friends for a dentist recommendation. (2) Check whether the first one takes your insurance. (3) If needed, check whether the second one takes your insurance. (4) Make an appointment. (5) Write it down on your calendar. See how that works? Can you text three friends today to ask if they have a dentist they like? That's a lot less intimidating than "deal with The Dentist." Write down each step and cross it off as you achieve it so you also have a sense of accomplishment along the way.

3

Find what's right with this challenge

One strategy that's easier than you might expect is recasting stress as gratitude, says Amit Sood, MD, executive director of the Global Center for Reliency and Well-Being, professor emeritus at the Mayo Clinic, and the author of *The Mayo Clinic Guide to Stress-Free Living*. "Relaxation is passive and doesn't give much for our mind to hold on to," he says. But gratitude is active—and it's correlated with feelings of satisfaction and joy. "Gratitude gives you access to positive emotions, which relaxation may or may not," says Sood. To try it, ask yourself, "What is right within what seems wrong?" Say you're nervous about your upcoming colonoscopy. What's good about it? You're fortunate to have access to a procedure that can keep you healthy. Or if you're feeling stressed about an overly booked social schedule, you might reflect on how thankful you are for your rich network of friends and remember the times they were there for you.

If possible, consider how your stressor might benefit

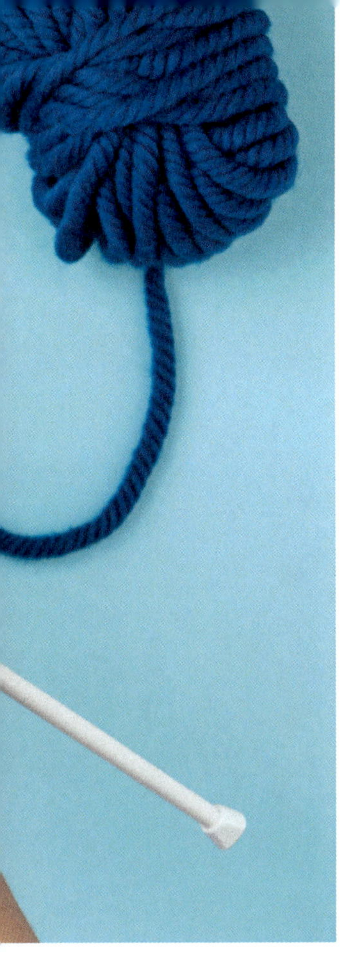

others. If planning a friend's baby shower is making you anxious, try to think about how much your efforts will ease her transition into parenthood and how grateful you are to help. "As you get into the nurturing mode, you release less of the stress hormone adrenaline and more of the bonding hormone oxytocin," says Sood.

4

Get (a little) angry

Anxiety is close not only to excitement on the scale of emotions but also to anger. (Think about that pounding heart or those sweaty hands.) Proceed with caution on this one: Too much anger can have toxic results, similar to too much unchecked stress, and approaching another person from a place of anger can be risky. But at the right time, you can channel your stress into productive anger, says Robertson, as long as you're able to regulate it without getting physically or verbally abusive. Say you're feeling anxious about a political or social injustice. Try turning the anxiety into righteous anger that will drive you to donate to a cause you care about or write to a politician.

5

Go to sleep

A good night's sleep can make a lot of things better, including stress. Shut-eye is an underrated anxiety fix, says Mary Alvord, PhD, psychologist and the author of *Conquer Negative Thinking for Teens*. When you're sleep-deprived, you get cranky, you can't think as clearly, and even small things can feel overwhelming. Research backs this up: A 2017 study published in the *Journal of Applied Psychology*, for instance, showed that employees were less likely to take out their work stress on their families when they got solid sleep (as well as plenty of exercise).

Of course, getting stressed and losing sleep can be a vicious circle: How do you fall asleep when you're already anxious? The first step, says Alvord, is to, well, not worry about it—when is the last time you truly never fell asleep? Try to stick to a regular bedtime schedule, even on the weekends. And avoid electronics for a good 30 minutes before bed—not just because of the now well-understood stimulating effects of blue light but also because consuming news can be too mentally stimulating right before sleep.

6

Redefine relaxation

What's "calming" for one person might not work for you. "These images of people relaxing on the beach—that's not relaxing for everybody," says Alvord. "Define relaxation for yourself." Maybe it's running outside, knitting, journaling, or binge-watching *The Marvelous Mrs. Maisel*. Figure out what feels right for you and know that it doesn't have to be an afternoon getting a spa pedicure.

When you find your happy place, make it a habit to revisit it regularly. That way relaxation is much less of a leap when you need it most. ●

"Ask yourself, 'Is there a problem here that I can solve? Would solving it lead me to less stress?' "

Finding the Right Therapist

SO YOU WANT TO WORK ON SOMETHING WITH A PRO. WE'LL GUIDE YOU THROUGH EVERY CONFUSING TURN OF THE MENTAL HEALTH MAZE.

By Andrea Petersen

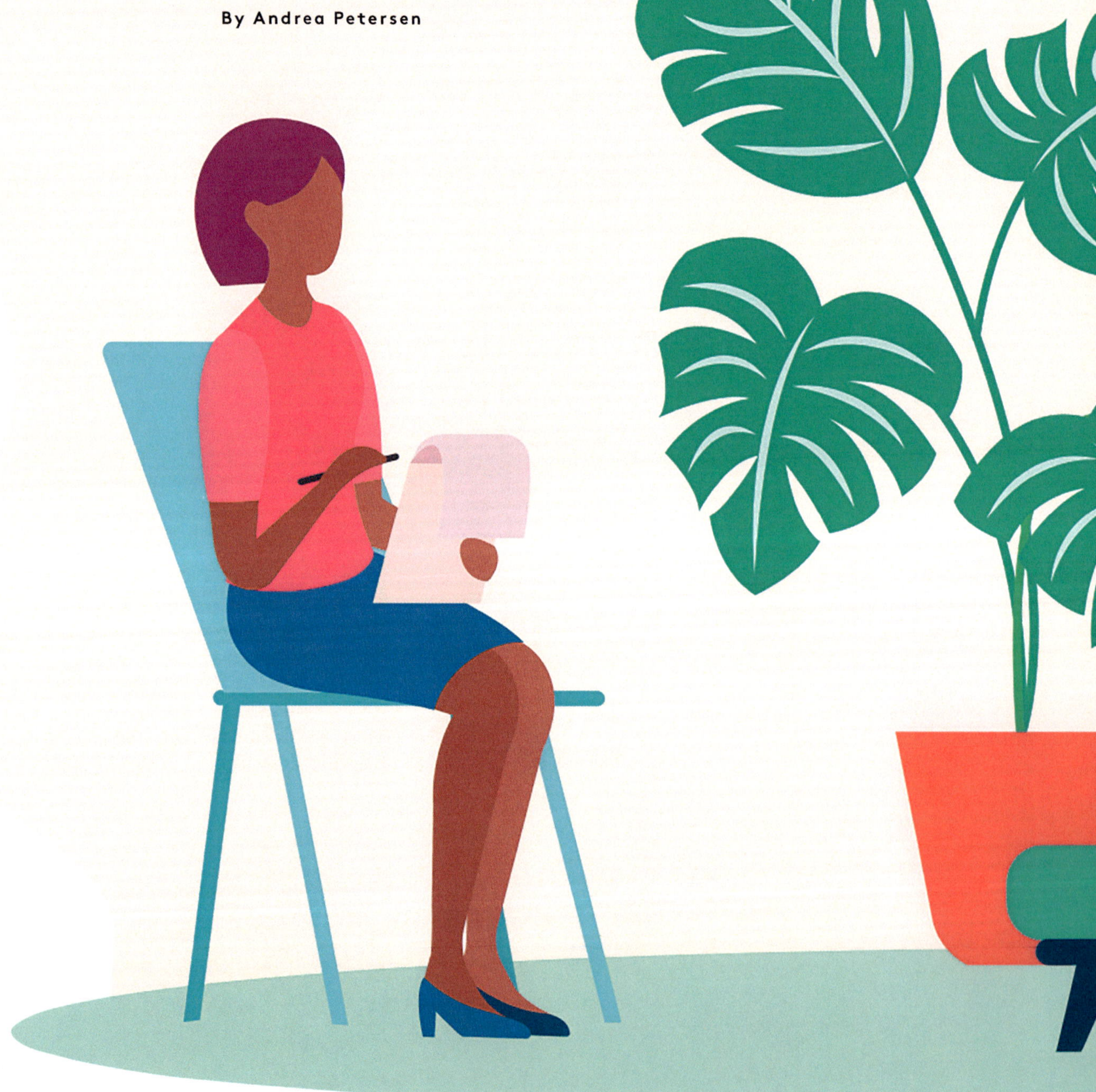

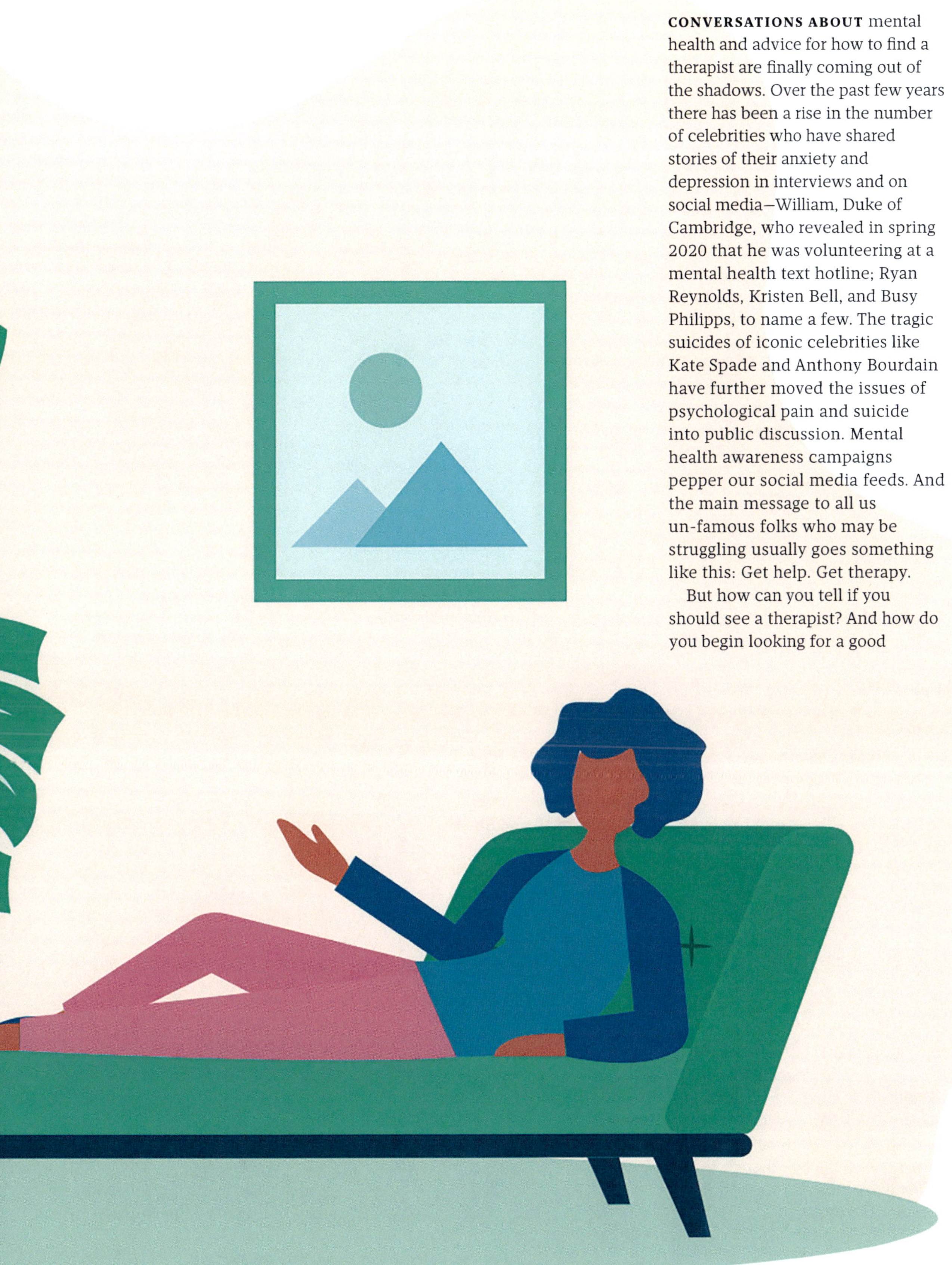

CONVERSATIONS ABOUT mental health and advice for how to find a therapist are finally coming out of the shadows. Over the past few years there has been a rise in the number of celebrities who have shared stories of their anxiety and depression in interviews and on social media—William, Duke of Cambridge, who revealed in spring 2020 that he was volunteering at a mental health text hotline; Ryan Reynolds, Kristen Bell, and Busy Philipps, to name a few. The tragic suicides of iconic celebrities like Kate Spade and Anthony Bourdain have further moved the issues of psychological pain and suicide into public discussion. Mental health awareness campaigns pepper our social media feeds. And the main message to all us un-famous folks who may be struggling usually goes something like this: Get help. Get therapy.

But how can you tell if you should see a therapist? And how do you begin looking for a good

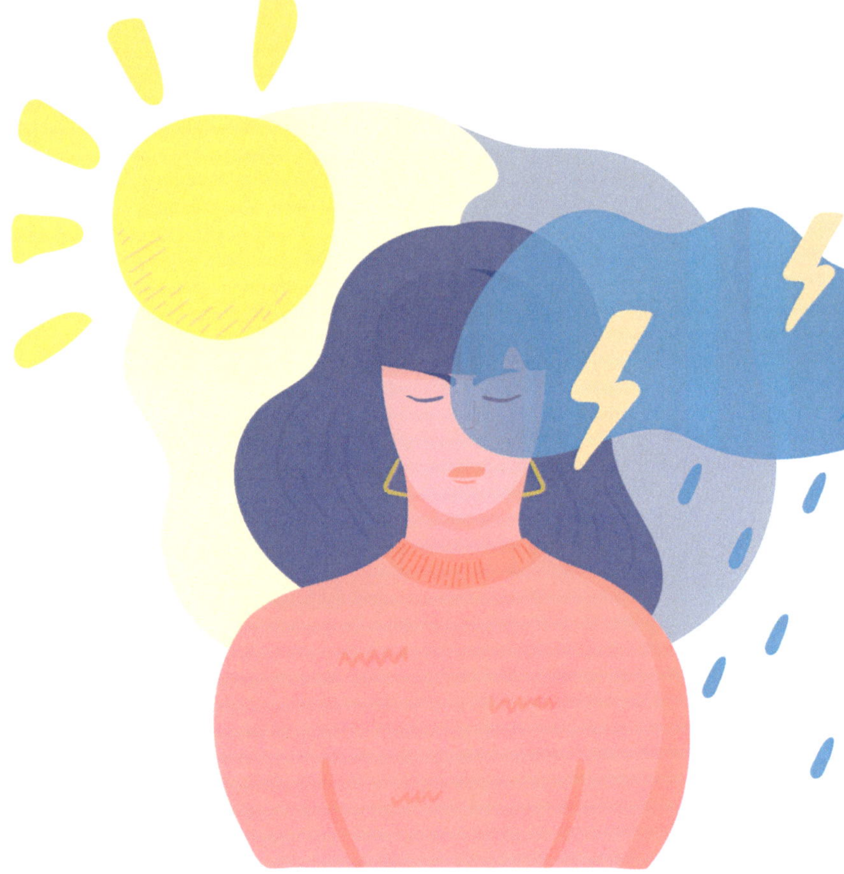

therapist who's ideal for what you're going through?

Unfortunately, finding the right therapist and treatment isn't always easy, especially if you're at an emotional low point. Google "psychotherapy" and you'll find a confusing alphabet soup of acronyms—ACT, CBT, and DBT, to name a few—for the various types of treatments. Even if you know what type of therapy you want, it can be hard to access it: 55 percent of counties in the U.S. have no psychiatrists, psychologists, or social workers, and sadly, many people don't get professional help at all. Only about 37 percent of those with anxiety disorders, for example, receive treatment, according to the Anxiety and Depression Association of America (ADAA).

The good news: If you do see a qualified therapist, chances are you'll find it helpful. Many talk-therapy treatments are backed by reams of rigorous clinical trial data. In fact, studies have shown that, for conditions like anxiety and depression, talk therapies are generally as effective as psychotropic medications, with fewer side effects and a longer-lasting impact. (That said, many patients benefit greatly from taking medication or from combining meds with therapy.)

Therapy isn't only for those who might be experiencing a mental health disorder. A therapist can help with relationship problems or challenging moments—say, a career shift or the loss of a loved one. Honestly, you may benefit from therapy if you simply need an objective person to talk to as a sounding board—especially if you're one to stew and let worries build up (or if you have no one else you can turn to at the time).

To get started in your therapist search, ask yourself what issues you want to tackle. Are you looking for guidance on a major life change? Or do you think you could be struggling with depression or another mental illness? You can find helpful glossaries on mental health conditions online from the American Psychiatric Association (APA), the ADAA, and the National Alliance on Mental Illness (NAMI). Then ask friends or your internist to recommend therapists that they think would be helpful. If you've had therapy before, consider what you liked about it—and what you didn't.

Find the right fit

The best therapist for you depends on your personal preferences, the convenience and cost of visits, and the provider's specialty or training (more on that below). Look for therapists who are members of a professional organization, such as the APA, ADAA, the National Association of Social Workers, or the Association for Behavioral and Cognitive Therapies. These groups offer continuing education and hold conferences to share research, so they are likely staying on top of advances, says Beth Salcedo, MD, the president of the ADAA and the medical director of the Ross Center in New York City and the D.C. area. Most of these groups' websites have databases that let you search for members near you—a great way to find practitioners.

How to interview a therapist

When you've found someone promising, request an informational phone call or a meet-and-greet before you dive into therapy sessions. Ask whether the provider has worked with other patients with your issues, as well as "how she would go about treating you, whether there's evidence for that approach, about how long it will take, and how you both will know when you're done," says Lynn Bufka, PhD, an associate executive director for practice research and policy at the American Psychological Association. If you're looking for someone with expertise in a particular type of therapy, ask how long their training lasted. (You may not want to see someone who completed only a daylong workshop.)

Ideally, you'll meet with a couple of therapists and pick the best fit. You should also feel confident about that provider's skills and comfortable with the idea of their challenging you, notes Bufka. And while you don't necessarily need to pick someone you'd want to be friends with, it is important that you feel you can be open with your therapist—and that they respect you.

What therapy costs

Some therapists use an income-based sliding-scale fee schedule. While most insurance plans offer some therapy coverage, many therapists don't take any insurance. To get coverage for those therapists, you need to have out-of-network benefits; you'll likely pay up front and then be reimbursed for whatever portion the plan covers.

Therapy is pricey—a session often costs $100 and up. But there are affordable options. Some therapists offer group therapy at lower rates. Community health centers often provide free or low-cost mental health services. Check out graduate psychology programs at local universities to see if there's a clinic offering treatment with a trainee.

Online therapy is another option. Companies like Talkspace and BetterHelp connect users with therapists through text, audio, and video chat. Aubrey Williams, of the Nashville area, started online therapy with Talkspace when she was struggling to get pregnant. She says she appreciated the price tag and the accessibility. "If I had a thought or a question at 2 a.m., I could just leave it for my therapist," says Williams. Studies have found that, in general, online therapy is about as effective as in-person treatment.

NAMI also has a help line (800-950-NAMI), and many local NAMI affiliates have free peer support groups. If you're in crisis, call the National Suicide Prevention Lifeline (800-273-8255). You absolutely don't have to let cost prevent you from getting much-needed help.

What type of therapy is best?

Your experience in sessions depends on the type of treatment—and many therapists combine multiple approaches. When considering practitioners, it's a good idea to ask which methods they use.

Cognitive behavioral therapy is the most research-backed treatment for anxiety disorders and depression. It's based partly on the idea that distorted thinking is a main cause of mental distress. Say you're in therapy for depression. If a friend didn't stop to chat at school drop-off, you might think, "She must hate me. I'm worthless." During CBT, a therapist would help you identify these unhelpful thoughts, challenge them, and replace them with more realistic ones ("My friend was probably busy"). For anxiety, CBT also usually involves "exposure," in which you gradually expose yourself to the thing you're afraid of. So if you have an elevator phobia, you'll work on feeling more comfortable in and near elevators.

If your therapist recommends acceptance and commitment therapy (ACT)—which research suggests is effective for anxiety, depression, and even chronic pain and substance abuse—you'll learn mindfulness techniques. (ACT is based on CBT but includes a strong focus on mindfulness and values.) ACT patients are taught to notice and accept challenging thoughts and feelings.

There's also dialectical behavior therapy (DBT), an in-depth treatment that combines CBT with other approaches and addresses suicidal and self-harm behaviors, borderline personality disorders, eating disorders, and substance abuse problems, among other issues.

What about meds?

Most therapists aren't allowed to prescribe medication. You'll usually need to consult a psychiatrist, your family doctor, or your ob/gyn for medications like antidepressants. If you think you would benefit from them, discuss it with your therapist, who can direct you to someone with prescribing authority. Ideally, the therapist and MD will work together to make sure you're getting the most appropriate care. ●

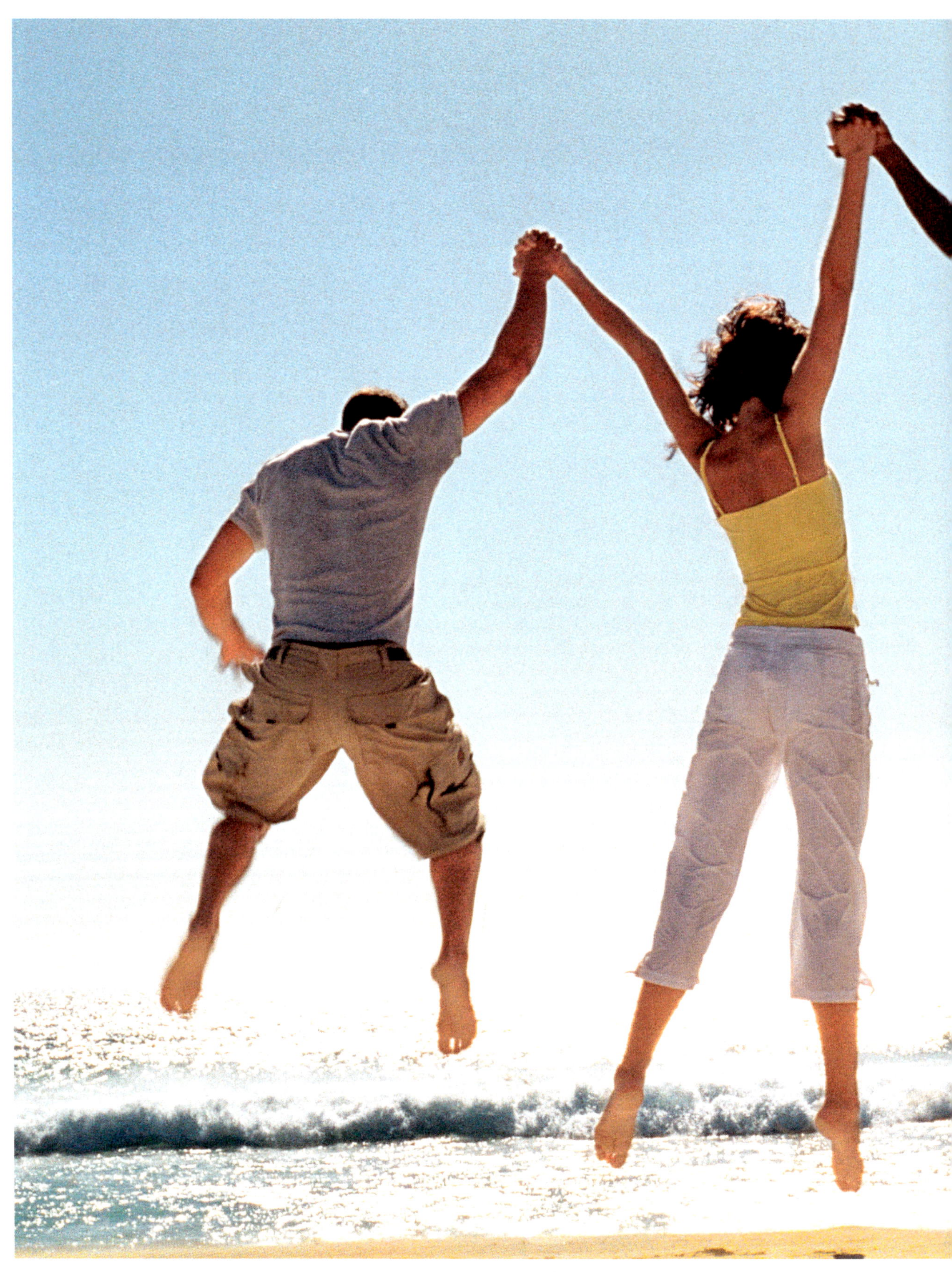

A Joyful Life

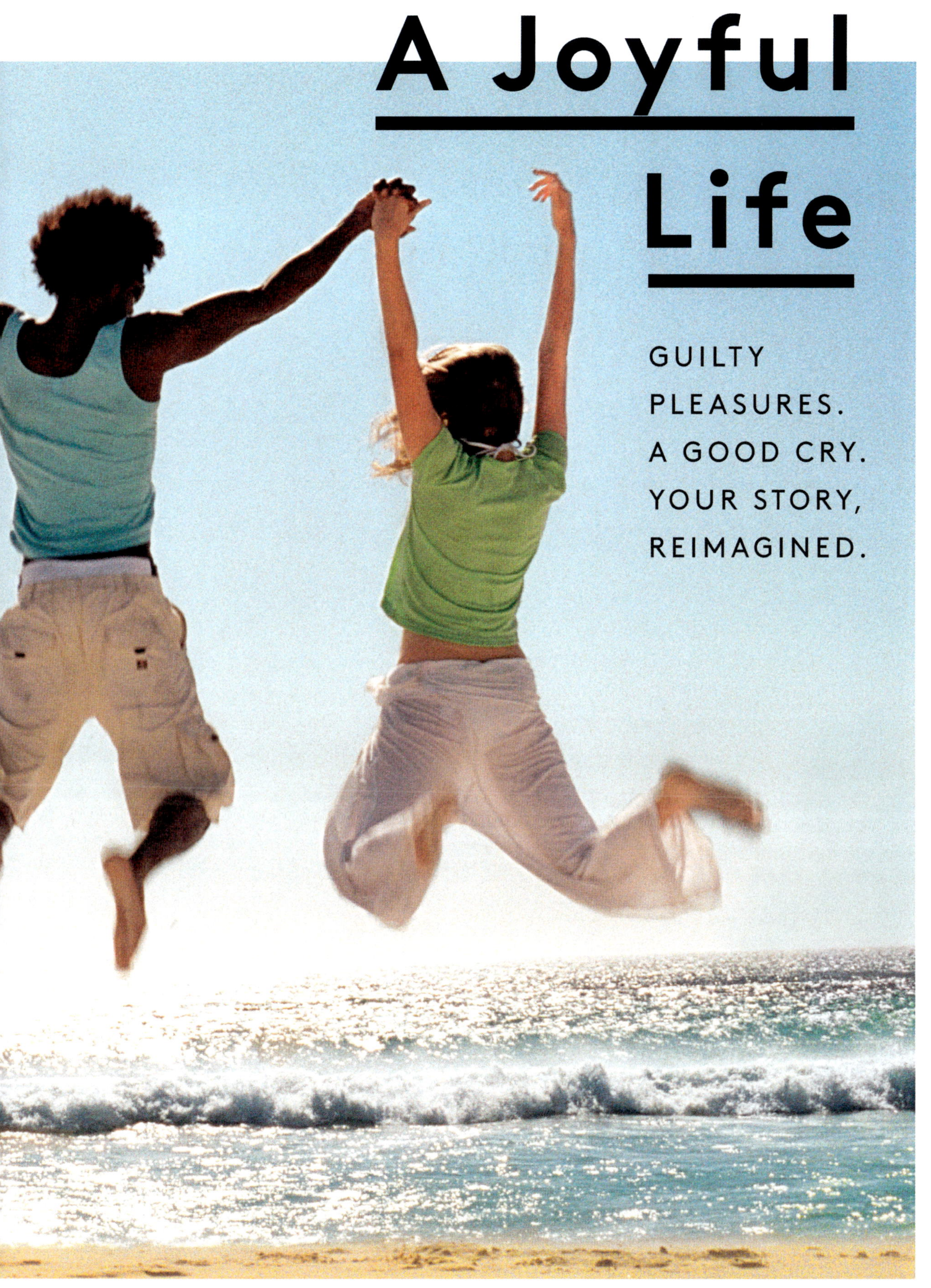

GUILTY PLEASURES. A GOOD CRY. YOUR STORY, REIMAGINED.

What I Do for Sanity's Sake When Nobody's Around

FROM A PRIVATE CANDY STASH TO A GUILTY STREAMING PLEASURE, WE ALL HAVE OUR QUIRKY WAYS TO ESCAPE THE GRIND OF MODERN LIFE.

By Janet Siroto

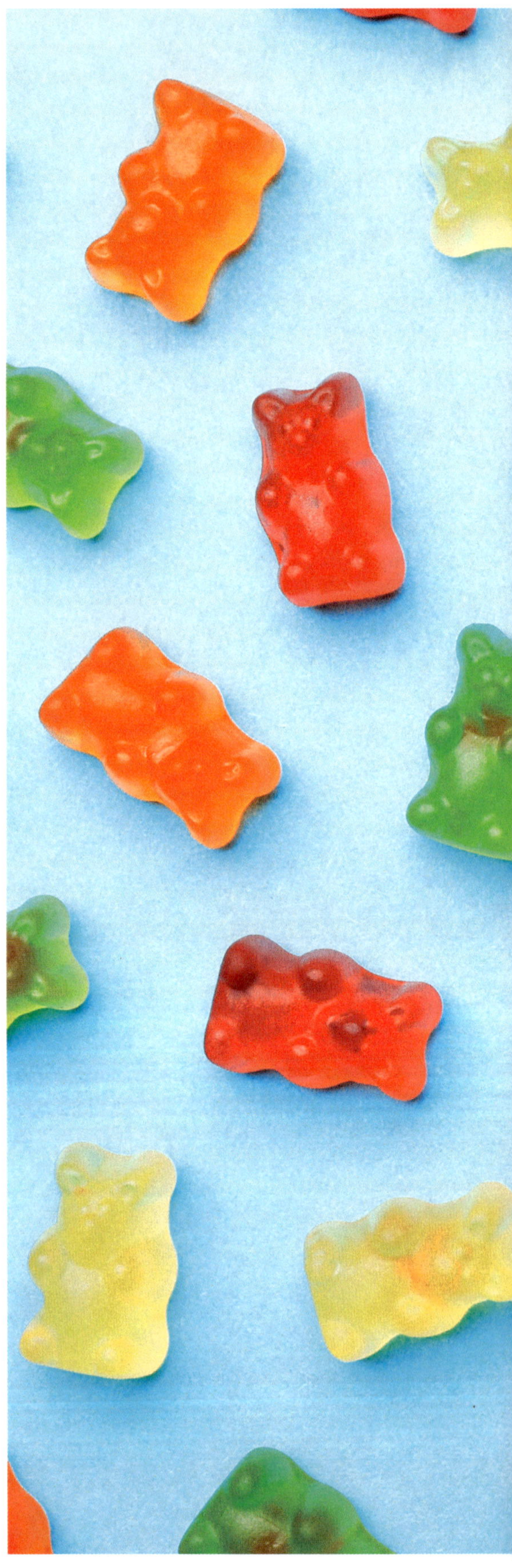

CONFESSION TIME: At the back of a kitchen cabinet, hidden behind the cornstarch and canisters of rice, far from the grabbing hands of my husband and kids, lies my secret stash, a jumbo resealable bag of Haribo gummy bears. While the label says "Party Pack," this party is for just one, thank you—me. I jokingly call these candies my stress-chew, because the delightful, almost rubbery texture really lets you chomp down with abandon. For me, eating them isn't about hunger; it's more akin to a dog working over a piece of rawhide. I usually dip into my supply when I'm feeling overloaded by responsibilities and random worries. ("How did I let us run out of milk? Why won't my boss reply to my urgent email, and is it too soon to nudge? Hey, when's my next mammogram supposed to be?") What's more, I eat them in a ritualistic order (face-

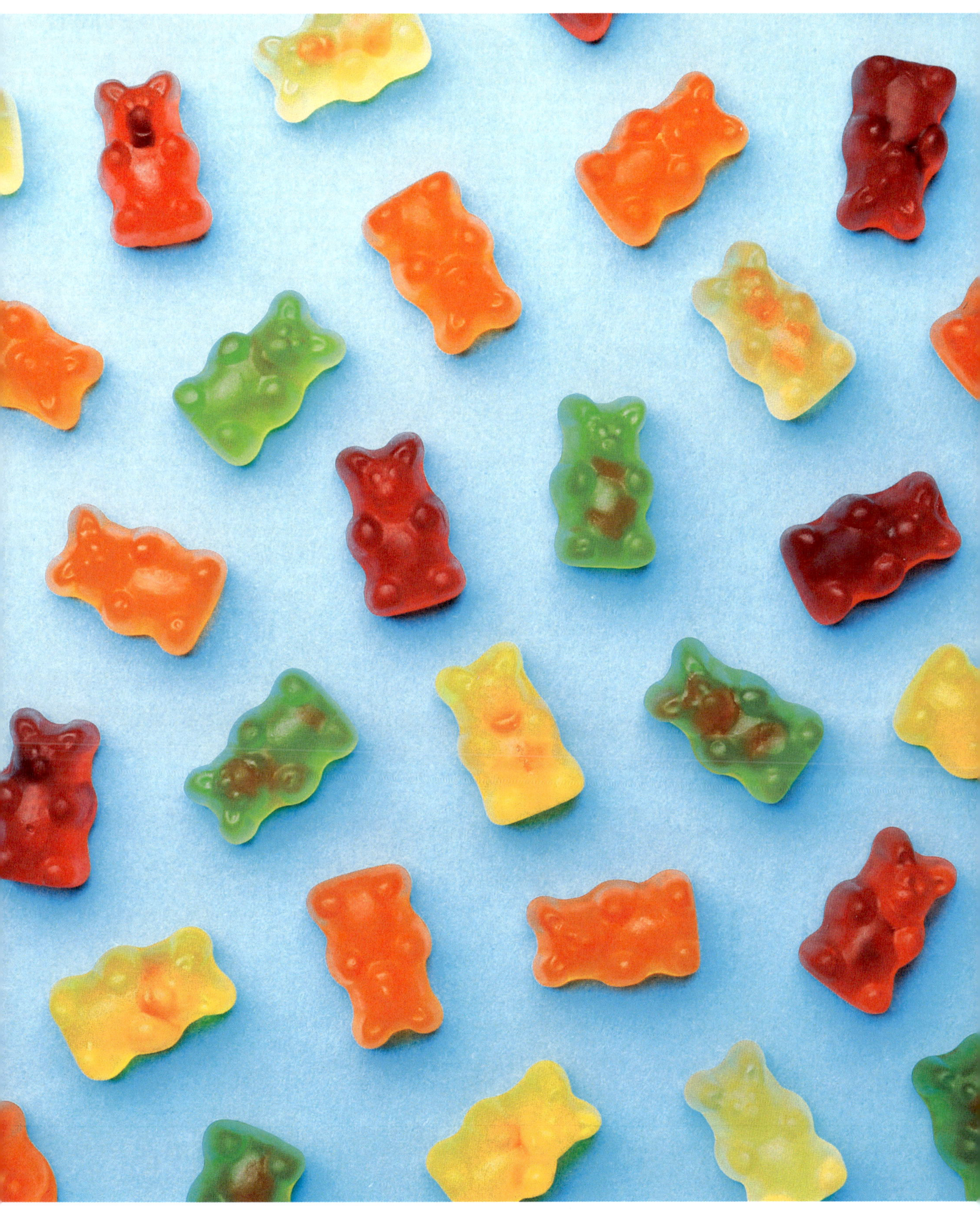

palm, but it's true): the less desirable yellows and oranges first, followed by red, then green, and then the jewel in the crown—clear pineapple—last. Part of their allure goes back to my happy memories associated with them. My mom used to buy me a small bag when she picked me up at elementary school at 3 p.m., and I'd joyfully tear through them on the way home. These candies are pure comfort, plus a sugar rush.

But if my dear husband were to catch me rooting around for my gummy fix? Oh, the shame!

A survey of friends and family tells me I'm not the only one with these weird, semi-mortifying rituals designed to self-soothe. We live in incredibly challenging times, with polls showing that our stress levels have been ratcheting up over the past decade to new highs, according to the *Gallup 2019 Global Emotions Report* (before the intensely stressful year of 2020 even hit!). Many of us have developed unique ways to calm ourselves the heck down—techniques that are far from the socially accepted practices of yoga and meditation. And we shouldn't feel ashamed of that, says Susie Moore, a Miami-based life coach and author.

"It's so funny that we women question our personal stress-relief strategies and feel shame around them: 'Am I doing this right? Am I doing this wrong?' There's no right or wrong way to live life or relieve pressure. It's about taking a break," she observes. "The only measure that matters is, 'Does this bring me joy? Does this calm me down?'"

But taking care of ourselves often feels like a nasty stew of laziness and self-indulgence. "American women in particular feel a massive amount of guilt around taking time for themselves," says Matthew Zawadzki, PhD, an associate professor of psychological studies at the University of California, Merced, and the director of the Stress and Health Lab there. "This is amplified by the demands of work, parenthood, and other forms of caregiving. Women feel as if when they do an activity, it has to be 'important.' Decompressing feels frivolous."

What's more, granting ourselves leisure time is good for our health. Zawadzki's research, published in *Annals of Behavioral Medicine*, has proven the value of ditching one's responsibilities for a while. "When people were doing what we call leisure, they were about 9 percent happier and 34 percent less stressed," he says, "and their heart rates were about 2.5 percent lower—an effect that lasted for at least an hour afterward, meaning less load on the body over time."

So if stress relief is such a good thing, why do we do it so stealthily? Secret rituals let us double-dip in tension taming: The activity itself lets us chill, and the fact that it's private means we can stay totally "in the zone," uninterrupted by other people's demands. For those of us who are major multitaskers (*umm*, just about all of us), it's heavenly to be in our own serene bubble of stress-busting bliss. For instance, if my husband saw me devouring gummy bears, he would want some. He'd probably want to chat, so I wouldn't be able to fully shut down my brain and enjoy mindlessly chomping on the springy little bundles of sugar. Part of what feels so good about these rituals is the withdrawal from "real life." As Moore puts it, "We all need to do a little more ball-dropping."

As it turns out, these covert tension-busters tend to cluster in a few categories. Each has its own way of boosting our ability to cope with modern life.

How creativity crushes the pressure

For many, quirky stress-relievers involve channeling creativity. Cortney Pellettieri, a cofounder of a talent-booking consultancy in Santa Monica, California, often feels tense from working with strong Hollywood egos and wrangling her three high-energy school-age children. "I wanted to do something creative to relax but needed to start in a low-stakes way. I ordered a bunch of paint-by-number kits. I pour a glass of wine, put on a podcast, and get to it. Yes, it's a total cheat, but I love it. I accidentally ordered one that's a bejeweled version called Paint with Diamonds. It has tiny pieces, and yet it wound up being a pretty relaxing pursuit that got me in the flow...but what

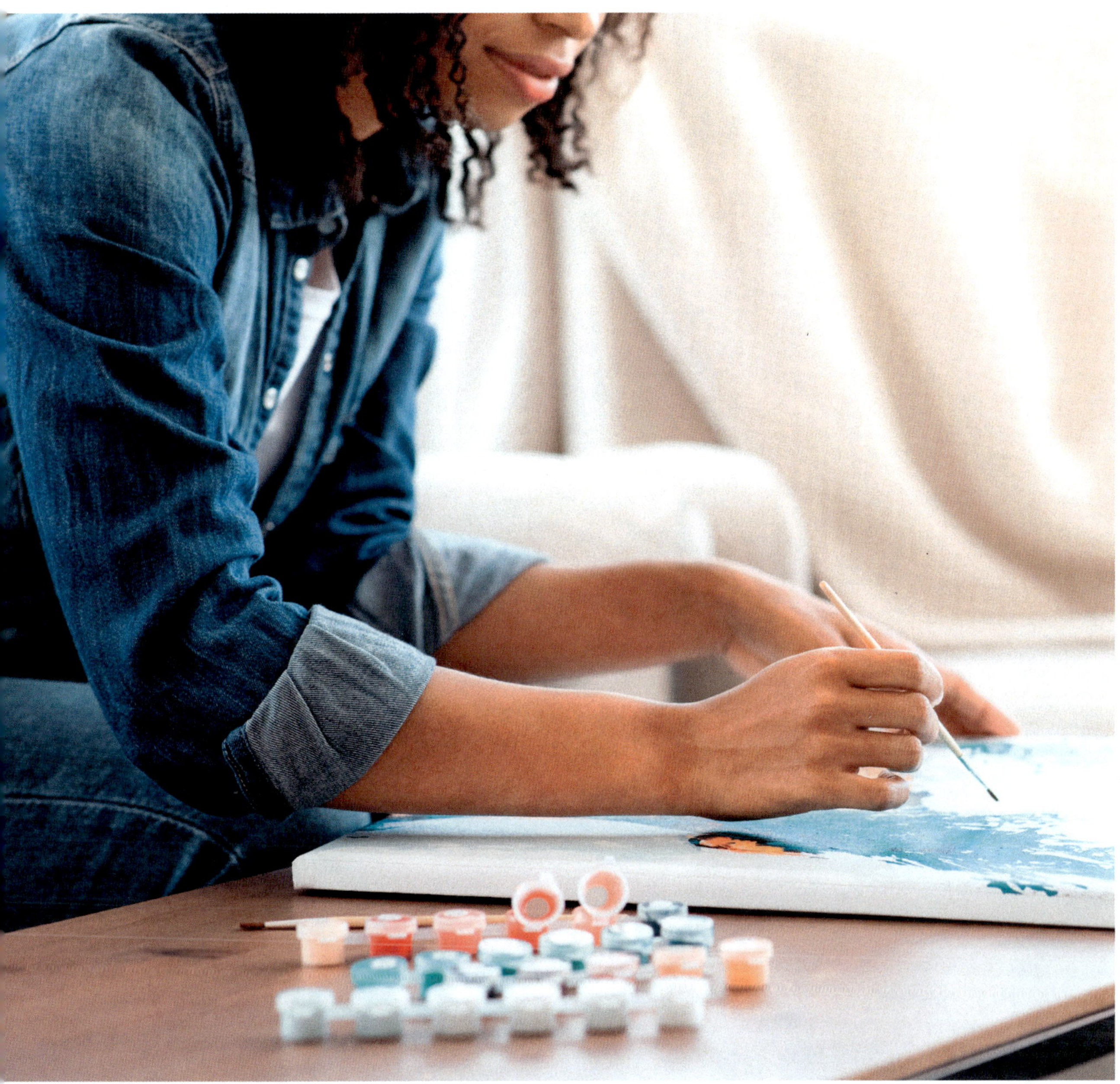

in the world am I going to do with bejeweled owl art?!"

Brooke Kosofsky Glassberg, an editor in Metuchen, New Jersey, has found a similar, slightly embarrassing way to chill. "I got into cross-stitching and am on my sixth needlepoint kit. I know it's not the coolest, most millennial hobby to have adopted, but it's really just another form of an adult coloring book. I find it extremely mindful and analog, both of which are key to getting through these days," she says. Projects like these can actually be the very best stress-busters, so there's no need for shame. Says Zawadzki, "Studies show that pure leisure—just lounging around—isn't as effective as active relaxation, something where you are absorbed in an activity. When you are in a flow state—feeling engrossed, competent, and challenged—you pull your mind away from ruminating. Research reveals you'll lower your blood pressure and be in a better mood. You are actively undoing your body's stress response." So what may feel like playtime is actually a beneficial act of self-care.

The rerun lovers' club

Another slightly mortifying way to decompress is watching "mindless" shows or cheesy movies that tend to

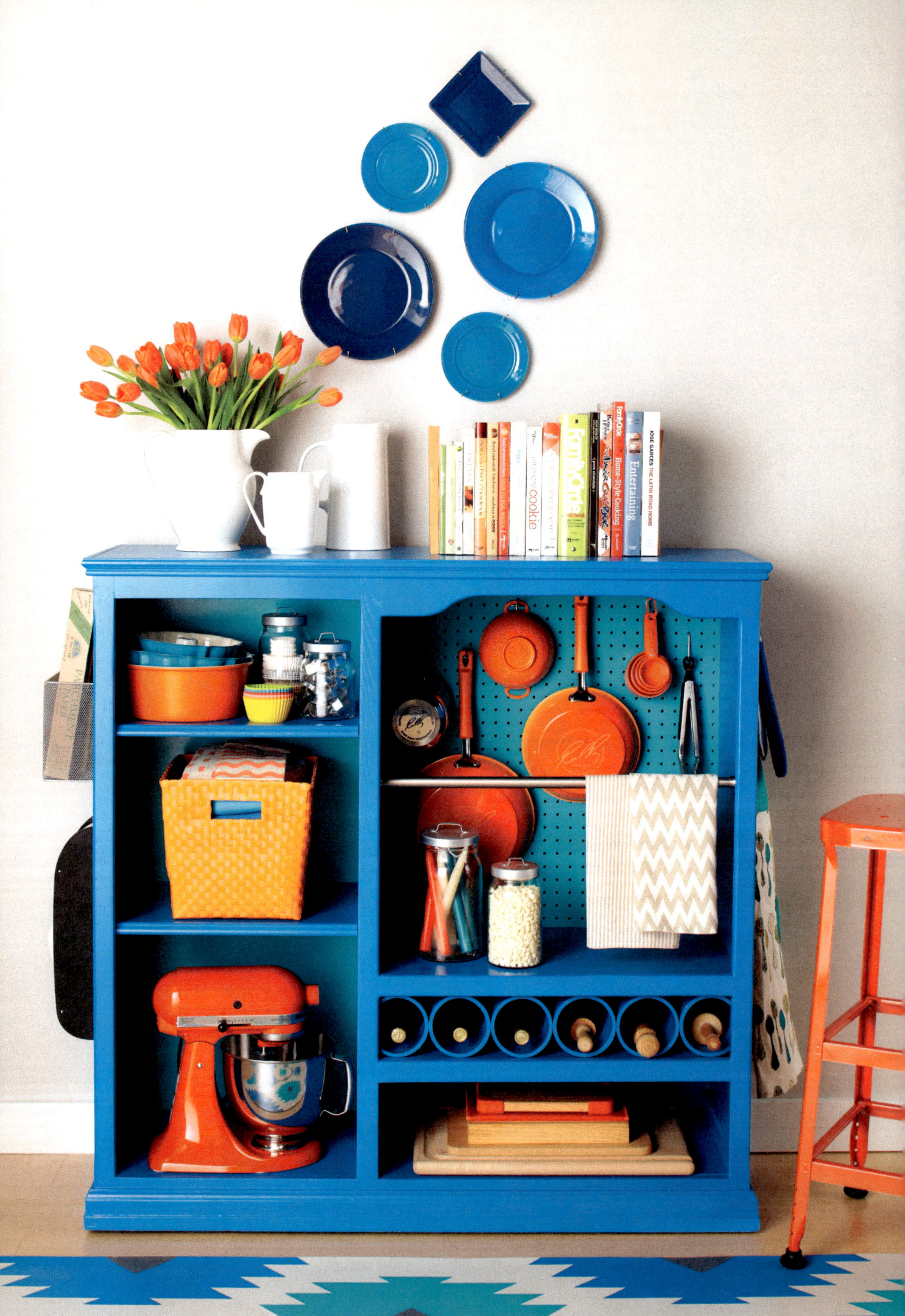
JOSE GARCES THE LATIN ROAD HOME
Entertaining
Home-Style Cooking
cookie

There's no harm in keeping these quirky rituals secret. As long as they're helping you cope with the intensity of your busy life and refilling your reserves, it's all good.

send other family members running from the room. I went through a *Real Housewives of New York* phase a few years ago that had my husband aghast. "What do you enjoy about watching these women shriek at and embarrass one another?" he'd ask. Good question! My answer was, "I may not live in a mansion, but I realize my life is better than theirs in some pretty key ways." A classic case of schadenfreude, a German term meaning "pleasure derived by someone from another person's misfortune."

But not all secret viewing has to have that train-wreck titillation. Rachel Bowie, a writer, editor, podcaster, and mom of a preschooler in Brooklyn, says her stress reliever of choice is a binge-a-thon of the show *Suits*, the series that happens to star Meghan Markle, now better known as the Duchess of Sussex. "My husband, Matt, is so eye-rolly about the show, so I watch it when he has a lot of work to do in the evening or when he's asleep, and I relish watching it alone," she says of her late-night reward. "I'm a major royal fan, so Meghan's scenes are for sure my favorite, but the whole show is the ultimate escape. I love the quippy one-liners and the fact that almost all the problems get solved by the end of the episode. Structure! Closure! It's all I want in my life right now."

This kind of chill-out time, while not elevating anyone's IQ or solving world hunger, can be vital. "Daily life often is full of obligations, and as humans, we struggle with our worthiness," says Moore. "We feel it's not OK to just take up space and do nothing—we must contribute! But enough—a lazy hour or day is OK." In other words, to do something that isn't productive is a very good thing. Everyone needs and deserves a break, and having your guilty-pleasure viewing is the perfect pastime.

The totally tidy obsession

It may seem counterintuitive, but some women turn to chores as their secret form of stress relief. More than a few of us can be found KonMari-ing ourselves into a drawer of beautifully folded, joy-sparking T-shirts. What's up with that? "Stress relief is something we do just for ourselves, to feel good, to feel calm. It makes your shoulders relax. It brings you joy," explains Moore. "For some people, that involves tackling an organization project. They get engrossed. They enjoy handling the objects they are sorting." Mindy Bianca, the founder of a PR agency for travel clients, can relate: "I'm always an 'everything in its exact place' person. So I was embarrassed that I have this one secret cabinet—a.k.a. the Cabinet of Doom—in my kitchen that has been a disaster. It was packed with recipes I'd torn out of magazines or printed out over the years... thousands of them. Completely out of control! It was like it was mocking me."

Bianca got "mega-gigantic binders" and plastic page protectors and dove into her project when she felt like she needed a break from work and everything going on in the world. "It gives me such a feeling of control to chip away at it," she notes, "and has reacquainted me with terrific recipes that, as I rediscover them, get added to my regular rotation."

Should your secret pleasure be, well, secret?

There's absolutely no harm in keeping your little comforts under wrap. As long as they are doing what they need to do—helping you cope with the intensity of your busy life and refill your reserves—it's all good. "If a private stress reliever brings joy, great! Enjoy the secret," says Moore. "The most important factor is how you feel. The last thing stress relief should do is generate more stress." Still, Zawadzki points out there may be an upside to letting your partner or a friend in on your little ritual. "We are social creatures," he says, "and there's something liberating about revealing these things to people we trust. It becomes a shared experience you can laugh at together. It helps us see that we fit in and are accepted"—quirks and all.

Which is great advice. But sorry, not sorry: The exact coordinates of my gummy-bear supply will remain hidden for the foreseeable future. ●

11 Life-Changing Lessons from TED Talks

THE IDEA-SPREADING NONPROFIT IS A MECCA FOR MENTAL WELLNESS ADVICE. BROWSE THIS CHEAT SHEET TO FIND INSIGHT AND INSPIRATION THAT FIT YOUR LIFE.

By Cassie Shortsleeve

IT USED TO BE THAT self-help was just the name of a bookstore aisle. Now we're as likely to tap into best-life advice through podcasts, YouTube videos, and TED Talks as we are reading best sellers. Want help with an issue big or small? Just search for it and you'll find someone somewhere with words of wisdom to share.

Technology makes it easy to work on ourselves on demand—no need to wait for a quiet time to sit down with your book. "A cellphone offers us endless opportunities to access self-help while doing other things, like cutting vegetables for dinner or sitting in traffic," says Dana Dorfman, PhD, a New York–based psychotherapist. With studies showing Americans are more stressed than ever, it's no wonder the most popular TED Talk videos on mental health have almost 50 million downloads each.

Want to explore life's big questions? Invite new perspectives into your life? Just find a few fresh stress-management tips? Here, top takeaways from some particularly enlightening TED Talks.

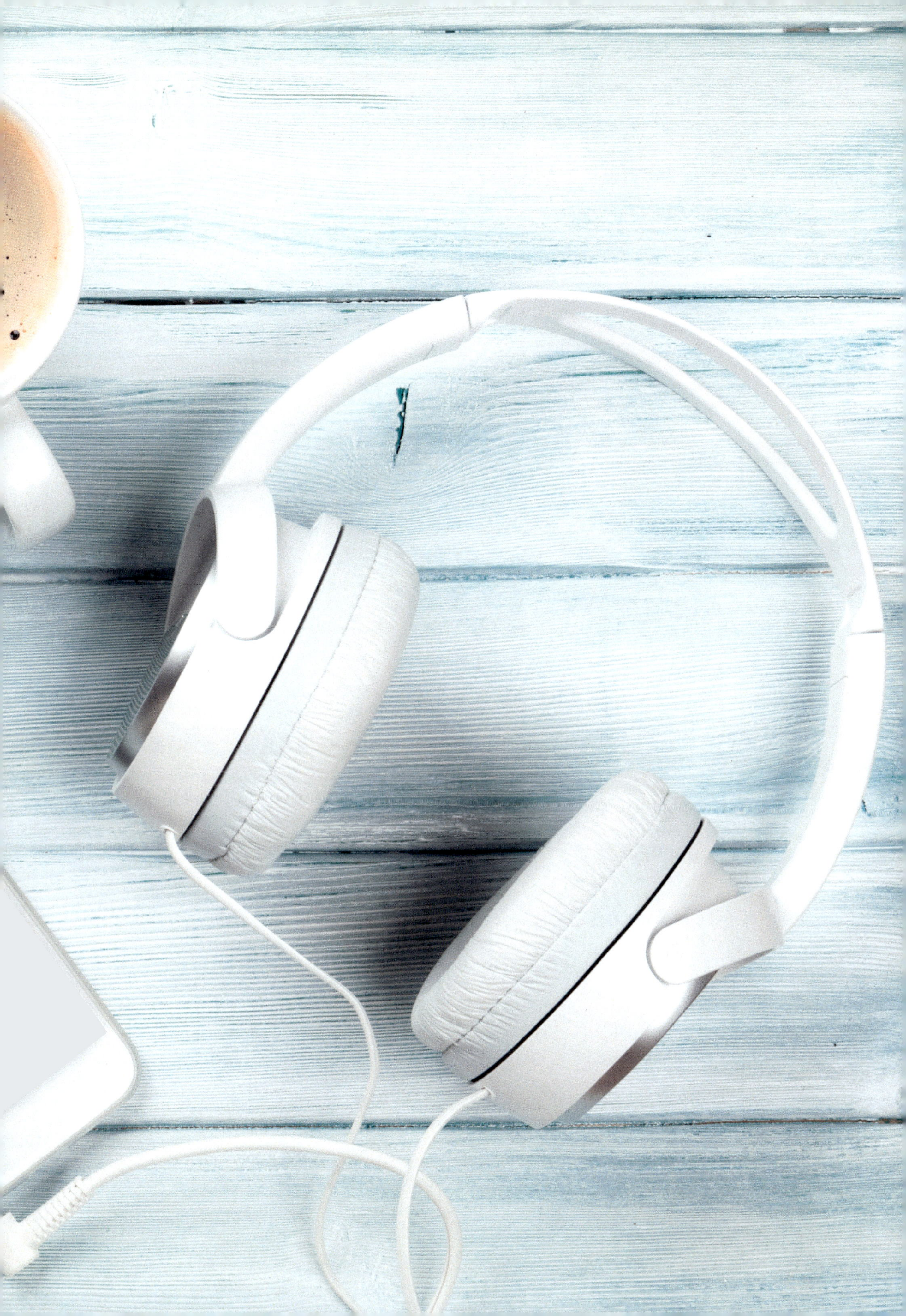

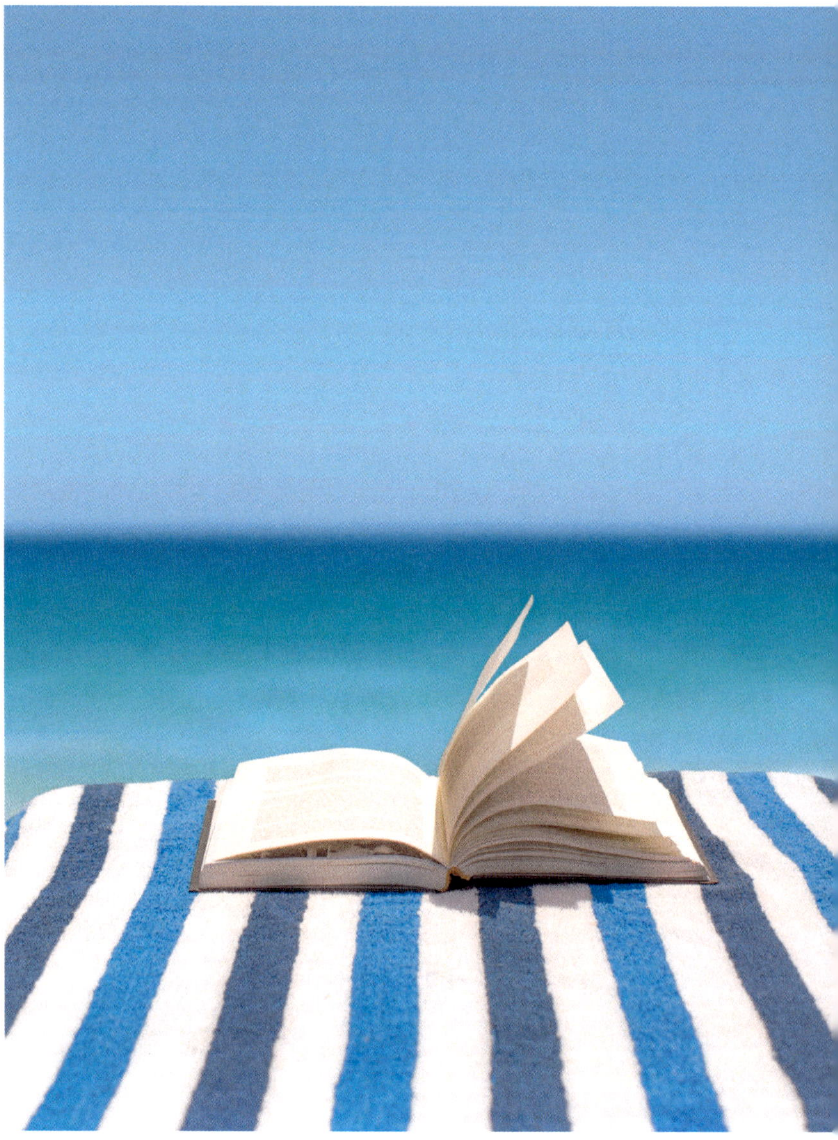

1

Be vulnerable

Years ago, professor Brené Brown, PhD, hated vulnerability. But in aiming to study shame, she unexpectedly stumbled on the discovery that "wholehearted" people—a.k.a. those who feel truly worthy—fully embraced the state. They put themselves out there. They were courageous. They were vulnerable. In her über-popular TED Talk "The Power of Vulnerability" (which has 48 million views), Brown details her struggles to accept—and live with—vulnerability and her discovery of its importance. The takeaway: Saying "I love you" first, doing something when there are no guarantees, and breathing through the uncomfortable aren't always easy. But let yourself be vulnerable. It's "the birthplace of joy, creativity, and belonging," Brown says.

2

Heal your mind with water

Wallace J. Nichols, PhD, a marine biologist and writer, loves the water. And he's not alone. For centuries, poets, doctors, artists, authors, and others have written about, studied, drawn, and detailed the healing powers of the sea. Think about it: How do you feel when you sit down on a beach or close your eyes and listen to waves crashing on a shoreline? In his talk, "Exploring Our Blue Mind," Nichols argues that water has the ability to temper stress, improve conversation, enhance creativity, and calm our minds. It helps us reach a peaceful state that he calls "blue mind," which is the opposite of a stressful, tech-filled mental state called "red mind." The best part? Even small, short exposures to water—a kayak ride, simply standing on the shoreline of a nearby sea—can help you feel calm. And it enables you to connect to yourself, the world around you, and others, which ultimately helps you find yourself in a busy, overstimulated world.

3

Delete the app that sucks your time away

When her son was born, the busy journalist Manoush Zomorodi was forced to spend hours walking around with him in a stroller just to get him to sleep. And she found herself bored. But she also realized that in those moments pushing the stroller, she had her most creative ideas. The experience led her to research the state of boredom and what it does to the brain. In "How Boredom Can Lead to Your Most Brilliant Ideas," she explains that being bored ignites the brain's default mode network (DMN) that helps you solve problems and form new neurological connections. Through intentional moments of boredom—deleting Instagram or Facebook from your phone for a day—you just might think outside the box more, notice more about the world around you, and finally figure out that issue that's been bugging you for weeks.

4

"In uncertain times think like a mother"

That's the name of women's-rights activist Yifat Susskind's TED Talk with more than 1 million views. The trick to facing crises head-on, she points out, is quite simply to think like a mom. (And, no, you don't need to be a mother to do it.) What exactly does "thinking like a mother" mean? "When you think like a mother, you prioritize the needs of the many, not the whims of the few," she explains. The takeaway: Next time you find yourself in a tough situation, try to recognize what others need, see yourself as the solution, and take action. It's something mothers do every day when they try to protect their children while also priming them for the best potential future possible (without ever knowing if what they're doing is truly going to make lasting, positive change). When you think about what others need—and take action to tackle a problem as best you can instead of waiting around to act—you can make progress toward your goals and solve issues that might otherwise grow to become even more problematic if left alone.

5

Find time for play

For one year, Shonda Rhimes, the creator and writer of hit shows like *Grey's Anatomy* and *Scandal*, decided to say yes to all the things that scared her: speaking in public, being on live TV, trying acting. She noticed that the very act of doing undid her fears. But in "My Year of Saying Yes to Everything," she notes that the one "yes" that changed her life the most was saying "yes" to playing with her three children every time they asked. What she realized? That play is the ticket to finding "the hum" of life—a.k.a. joy, confidence, and peace. Rhimes wound up making it a rule that she would always agree to play with her kids. But your "play" could mean doing anything that makes you feel good and free and happy—even for 15 minutes. "Want to play?" should mean giving yourself a few minutes of indulgence.

6

Spend three minutes a day in silence

In his talk "5 Ways to Listen Better," sound expert Julian Treasure argues that, as a society, we're losing our ability to listen. And that's not just because the world is a loud place and that listening

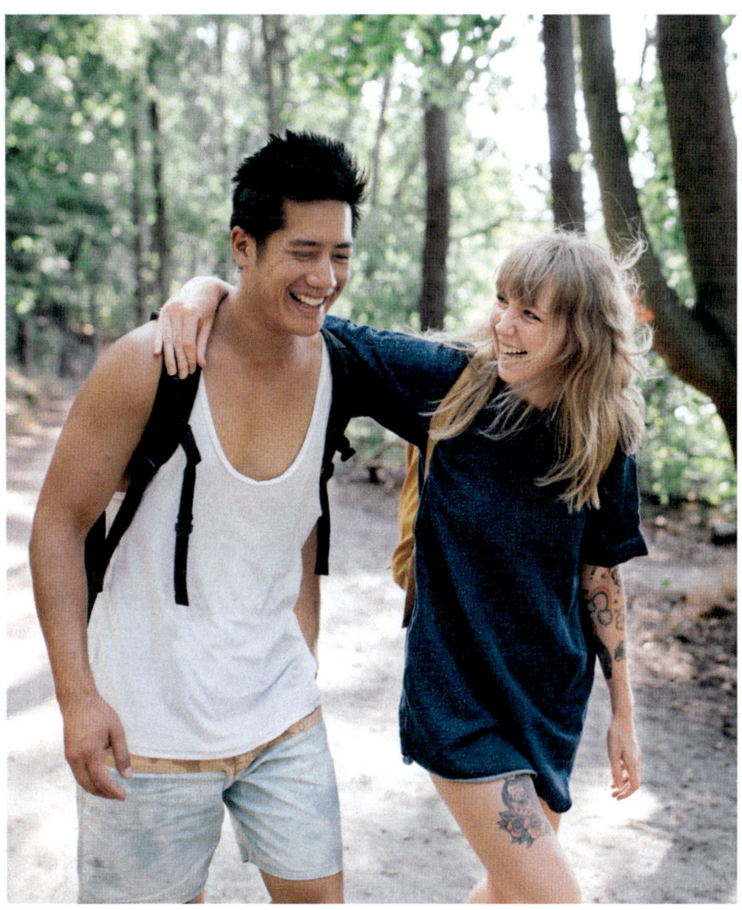

is tiring, but also because we're becoming headphone-wearing personal broadcasters who have no space (mental or physical) to truly listen. It's a problem, he explains, since listening is our access to understanding—and when we become desensitized by noise, it becomes harder to pay attention to the quiet and the understated. One suggestion he offers to enhance your listening: Spend three minutes in silence each day to reset your ears and recalibrate you so that, as he says, "you can hear the quiet."

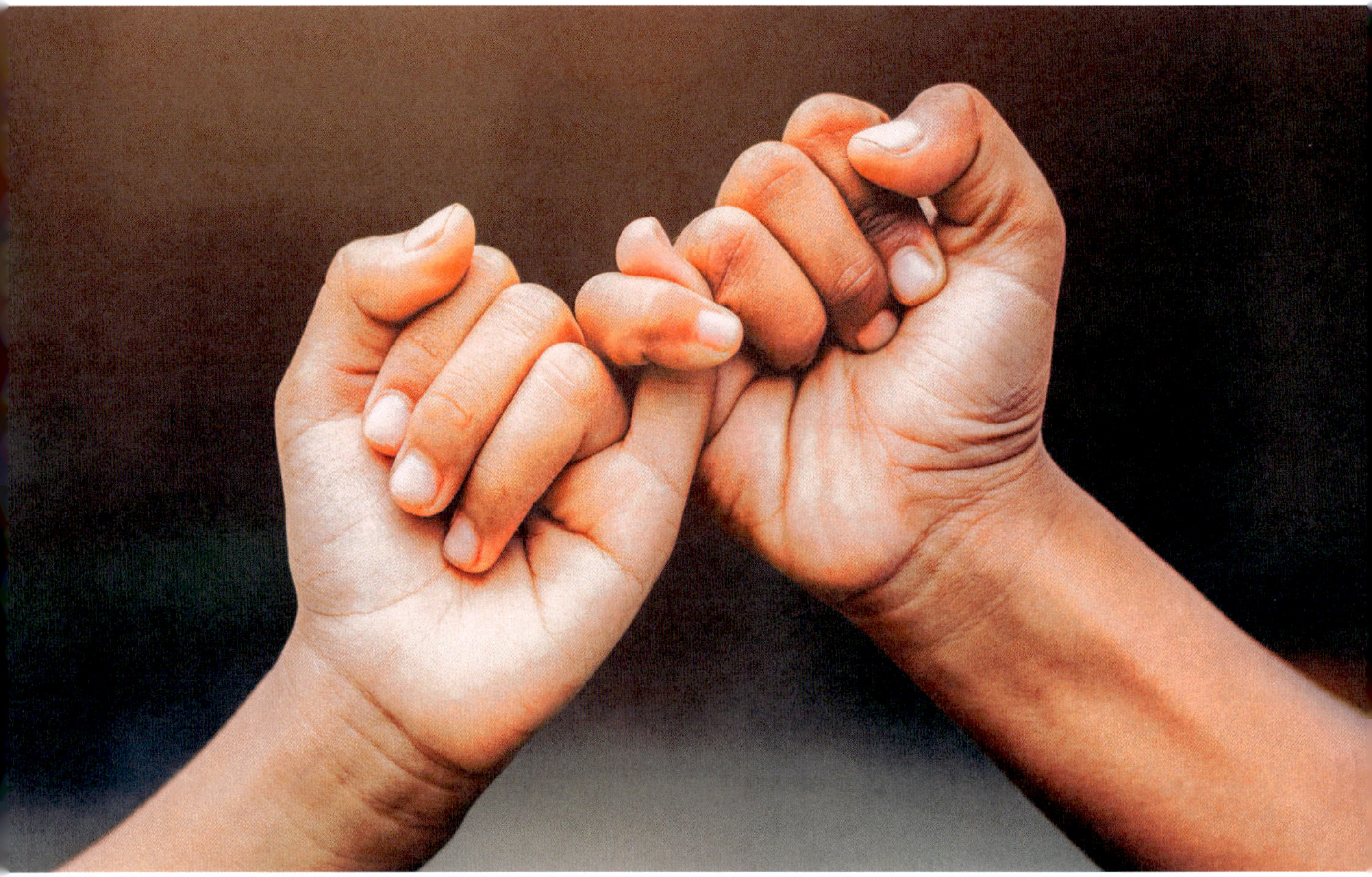

7

Tend to friendships for a long, joyful life

Most people want to get rich and find "success" in life. But are those the things that generate happiness? Not quite, points out Harvard psychiatrist Robert Waldinger, MD, the director of the Harvard Study for Adult Development—arguably the longest study of its kind, which began tracking the lives of 264 Harvard sophomores 82 years ago (and now their 1,300 offspring) to find out what brings happiness throughout life. In the TED Talk "Lessons from the Longest Study on Happiness," Waldinger reveals that good relationships keep us happy and healthy. Social connections, it turns out, are vital for well-being—and the quality of relationships matters more than the quantity. In fact, the men who were the most satisfied with their relationships at 50 were the healthiest at 80. In short: Keeping up close ties has the power to buffer us from aging-related health and mental health issues.

8

Talk about race even—and especially—if it's uncomfortable

Finance executive Mellody Hobson knows that race isn't always easy to talk about, and in her TED Talk "Color Blind or Color Brave," she does just that, pointing out in 2014 what our society has only recently been waking up to: the fact that we need to face topics that make us uncomfortable head-on and learn to be comfortable with the uncomfortable. She stresses that "color blindness" is dangerous—it means we're ignoring the problem. Instead, being "color brave"—willing to have proactive conversations about race with honesty, understanding, and courage—is the solution. "Invite people into your life who don't look like you, don't think like you, don't act like you, don't come from where you came from," Hobson says, "and you might find that they will challenge your assumptions and make you grow as a person."

9

Beat stress by reaching out

You've likely heard that when the stress hormone cortisol is chronically elevated, it ups your risk of disease, hinders your mental health, and hurts productivity. But in her talk "How to Make Stress Your Friend," health psychologist Kelly McGonigal, PhD, notes that oxytocin—a.k.a. the "cuddle hormone"—is also a stress hormone. The pituitary gland releases it as part of the stress response. Oxytocin primes you to take action, connect, and strengthen close relationships. In fact, it even helps your heart heal from stress-related damage. "Your biological stress response is nudging you to tell someone how you feel instead of bottling it up," she says. So the next time you feel stress rising? Reach out to others for support. Or connect to help someone else, which is healthy for both parties. One five-year study following nearly 1,000 adults found that after enduring a stressful life event like a job loss or a death in the family, the folks who regularly helped others were less likely to die than those who didn't. In the presence of human connection, your stress response will become healthier and you'll recover from stress more easily.

10

Remember: Happiness isn't a destination

Most people think that winning the lottery, getting a promotion, or finding true love will bring happiness. But that's not exactly the case. The truth is, these things don't make us joyful for long. And humans have a "psychological immune system" that allows us to be happy even when things don't go our way, Harvard psychologist Dan Gilbert, PhD, details in his popular TED Talk "The Surprising Science of Happiness." Even more, knowing that you have this ability can be a benefit, helping you experience even more happiness no matter what you're facing. Studies suggest this "synthetic happiness"—in other words, what we settle for when we don't get what we wanted—is just as satisfying as "natural happiness," which results when a dream comes true. It's all good news, because it means we're more resilient than we may think.

11

Be kind to yourself after heartbreak

At some point, most of us face heartbreak, and since losing love creates dramatic and, in fact, physiological pain, many people have a hard time getting over it, psychologist Guy Winch, PhD, explains in his TED Talk "How to Fix a Broken Heart." Fortunately, he shares strategies to move on in a healthy way. First? Remember all the ways in which you and your former partner were wrong for each other—and keep that list on your phone. By not "going down memory lane," you avoid idealizing the relationship and staying stuck in the past. Also think about the voids that your lost relationship has left in your life, including social voids, voids in identity, even physical voids in your home. Working to fill these empty spaces helps you re-establish who you are. ●

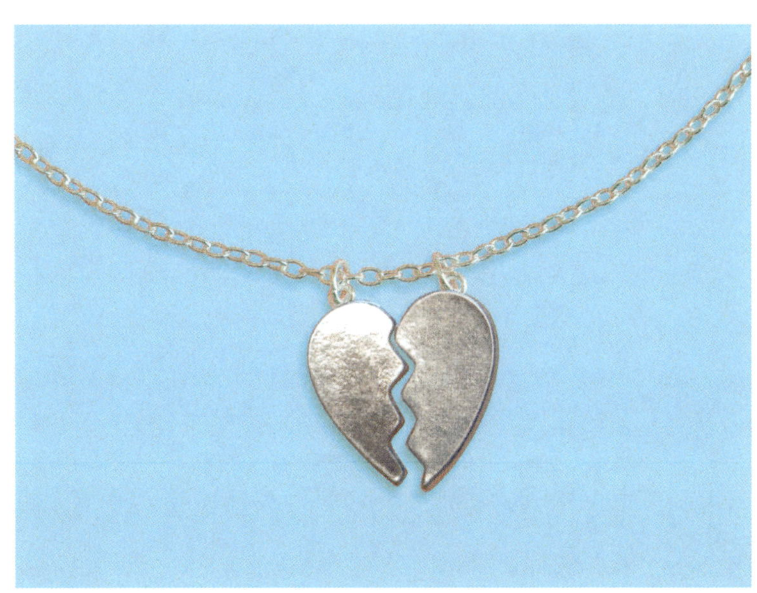

Cry It Out

LEANING INTO YOUR TOUGH EMOTIONS IS AN UNEXPECTED SECRET TO REAL JOY.

By Lisa Lombardi

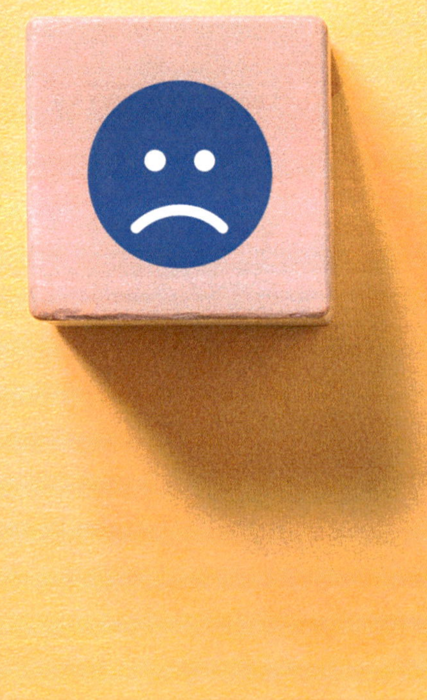

A FEW YEARS AGO, I had one of those days when everything goes epically wrong. A doctor told me I needed a biopsy—of my eye. The babysitter called to say water was running into our just-renovated basement. I raced home to get my son ready for his orchestra concert and couldn't tie his tie...but also: I needed gas. So I left him in tears to go to the gas station, only to run over the island and blow out my tire. Later, as I listened to the soothing sound of strings in the dark auditorium, my mind drifted to my ruined basement and weird health scare and all I wanted to do was hurl myself on my bed like a 14-year-old and sob at the unfairness of it all.

Is there a case for wallowing in self-pity? We're taught to count our blessings, say namaste, and move on. But sometimes you want to first feel what you're feeling: *Waaah.* As counterintuitive as it sounds, leaning into the tough stuff is good for us. "Feeling bad is something that has actually evolved to help us to thrive," says Susan David, PhD, an instructor in psychology at Harvard Medical School and the author of *Emotional Agility*. "Our full range of emotions helps us signal to other people things like we need help or we're scared. And they help us signal to ourselves that something important is at stake."

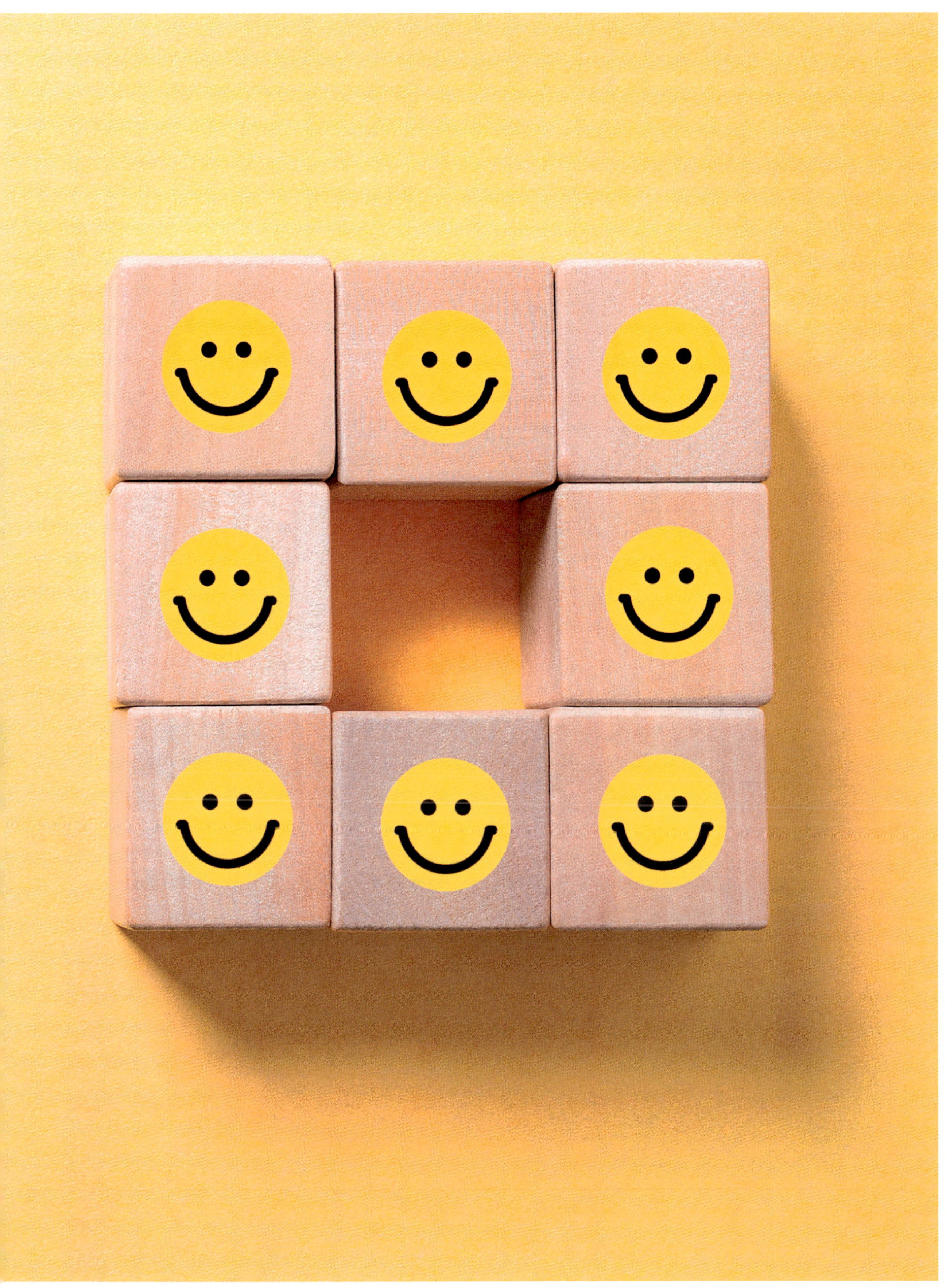

A good cry

Crying also serves a purpose: It feels cathartic because it truly is. "Crying is a kind of release," explains Alicia Walf, PhD, a senior lecturer in cognitive science at Rensselaer Polytechnic Institute in Troy, New York. Whether we tear up a little or full-on wail, the act of crying helps us recover from challenging emotions like sadness, fear, and anger (as well as intense positive ones like happiness and awe). "There's a fair amount of research showing that crying evokes a kind of calming neurological effect that allows us to begin the process of releasing and self-soothing," says David.

You just may have to wait a beat. In a study published in the journal *Motivation and Emotion*, researchers had people watch a tearjerker. Half cried, and half didn't. At first, the criers' moods dipped, but when researchers checked back after 90 minutes, the criers felt sunnier than they had before the film started, while the non-criers reported no mood boost.

Both emotional crying and the tears you get from cutting an onion come from the eyes' lacrimal glands, but similarities between the two end there. "There is literally a difference in the tears from emotional crying and the ones you get from hurting your eye," says Walf. The emotional tears contain neurotransmitters and different protein levels than the dry-eye type tears. And they're stickier, which means you can see them on someone's face. That means your sad or angry tears let everyone around you know—and you know too—that you're experiencing some pretty major emotions.

In fact, emotional tears happen on a brain level. "Our emotional tears involve different circuits that are related to our emotional brain, our limbic system, and our stress response," Walf explains. Crying—whether it's over a breakup, a sad episode of *This Is Us*, or the final straw on a day from hell—triggers a stress response, with the same kind of increases in heart rate and blood pressure you get from other challenges to the body. "It's like your body is telling you, 'These are intense emotions,'" Walf says.

And here's a fun fact: Most infant animals do some kind of distress calling, but we're the only creatures that continue to cry this way as adults.

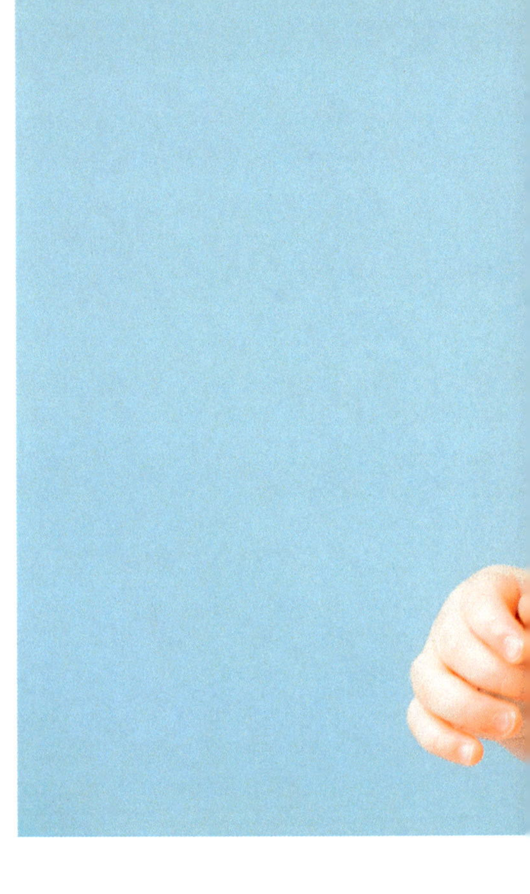

Crying helps us recover from challenging emotions like sadness, fear, and anger.

Human babies make crying sounds from birth onward, but it isn't until around 4 to 8 weeks of age that they put together distress calling with physical tears, Walf says. (If you never realized that your newborn wasn't shedding tears for the first few weeks, you're not the only one!) Wailing is a way for tiny, vulnerable infants to get what they need and start to bond with their caregivers.

You may have noticed that some people don't cry at all (no, they're not sociopaths—it's normal!). On average, women cry twice as much as men, tearing up about two to four times a month. "But there are

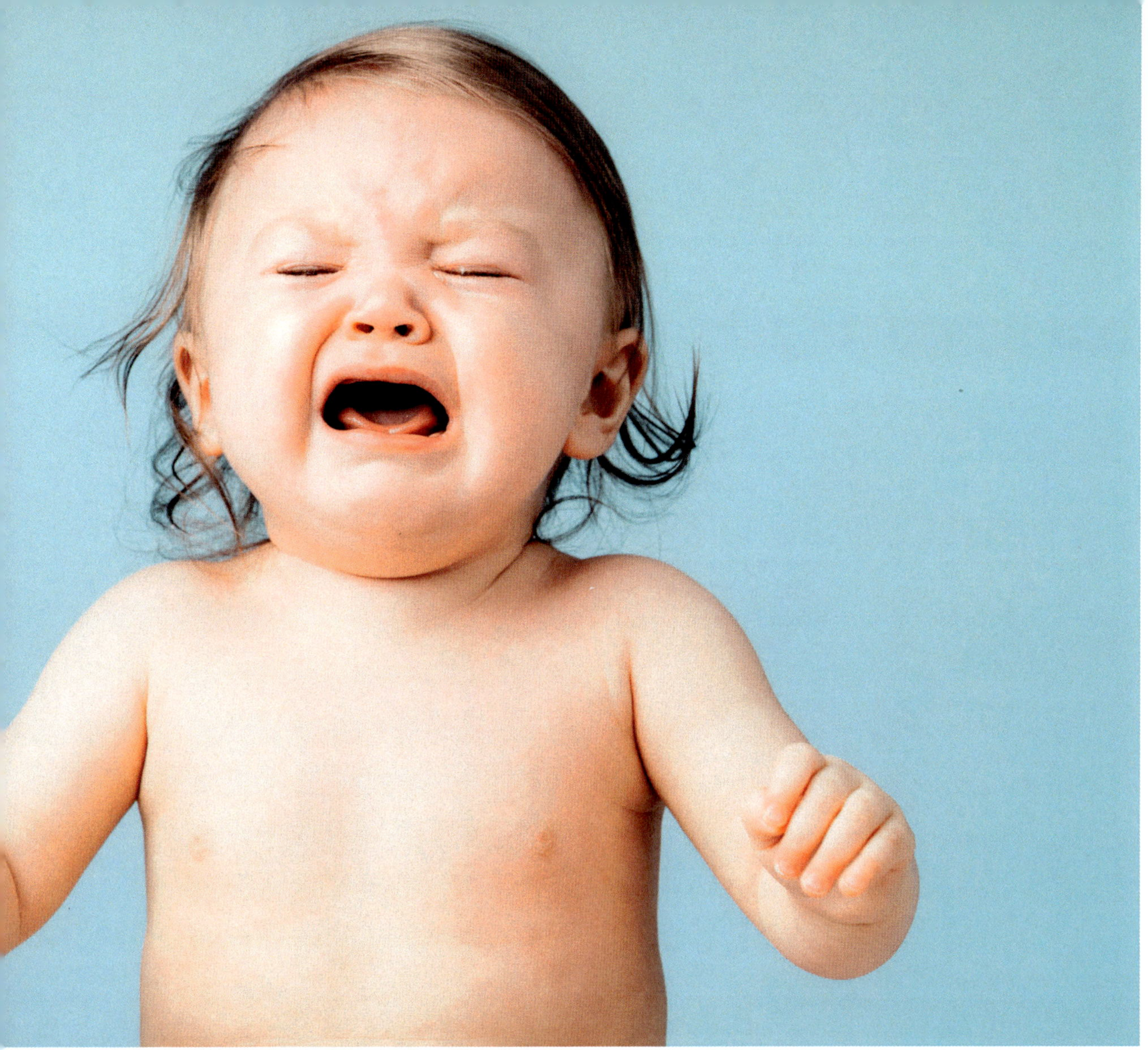

non-criers and super-criers," Walf stresses—so the average numbers may not mean much.

We cry to communicate we're in need and vulnerable. And if we're in imminent danger, we sometimes signal this by tearing up without making a sound. Why? "One thought is this is helpful in a safety way: You're telling someone 'Something's wrong, I need your help' without alerting the predator," Walf explains. We also do the opposite, bringing up the sounds of wailing but not the waterworks.

The upside of down moods

While difficult emotions don't always lead to tears, they often make us feel uncomfortable. But boredom, anger, sadness, guilt, and other so-called bad emotions are there to help. They provide the "emotional data," as David calls it, to move our lives in a direction that will make us happier. Still, we get bombarded with the message that we should feel chipper all the time. We hear it from family and friends, Instagram posts, and even bosses and coaches. It's part of our American culture and history, after all. The pursuit of happiness is right in the Declaration of Independence, David points out. "When we grow up in a culture which says be positive, no matter what's going on—you can be diagnosed with cancer and it's 'Just be positive'—what happens is you start to layer on unhelpful emotions," she says. So you feel sad about being sad or stressed about being stressed. You think, "Oh no, I'm the saddest person I know on Instagram." Or you worry, "All this nonstop worrying is going to give me an autoimmune disease." The upshot: You end up feeling even worse.

Instead, experts say to think of your tough emotions as clues, there to help you identify what's not making you happy in your life. Once you recognize the trouble areas, you can take some concrete steps to get to a happier place, one that aligns more with your values.

So next time you feel sad or annoyed, say, note exactly what you're feeling and dig to figure out the root cause. Let's say you feel cranky after work. Instead of pushing the feeling away, ask yourself, "What's going on here?" You might realize you're annoyed because your new boss undermines you in meetings. If you ignore the initial sadness, you miss the message—and the chance to change your situation for the better by talking to your manager about your frustrations or working on your résumé so you can get the heck out of there.

David advises we ask ourselves, "What is the situation? And what is the values-connected response to the situation?" Considering your values lets you decipher the data and use it to change your life for the better. So in the annoyed-after-work scenario, maybe you value respect and you work in a toxic environment. You value doing good for others, and your company defends toxic dumping. By mulling over your funk, you might realize you'd rather be a lawyer for a nonprofit with a work-friendly culture. Or that you'd like to take on pro bono cases on the side to help others.

This is all part of what David calls emotional competence. You'll know you have it if "you're open to your emotions and you experience and understand them. And you use emotions in the way they were intended, which is to help you to adapt and thrive and be authentically happy, rather than a forced and false pursuit of this supposed thing you're meant to be," she says.

Developing emotional courage

The problem is, many of us spend our energy trying to tamp down or distract ourselves from our darker emotions, whether we realize we're doing it or not. And if you grew up in a family where every time you had a terrible day at school, Mom or Dad would chirp, "Hey, who wants a big bowl of ice cream?" then you might be particularly prone to bottling the sadness and the outrage. The other big mistake many of us make is brooding, which is ruminating and dwelling—feeling sad about being sad. (See: my self-pity-induced bed flop.) There's good reason to avoid these coping methods: Both styles are linked to higher levels of depression, high levels of anxiety, lower levels of well-being, and more difficulty in relationships.

If you ignore your sadness, you miss the message—and the chance to change your situation for the better.

David explains that one way to understand brooding and bottling is to imagine that your negative emotion is on a piece of paper. The bottler crumples and tosses the paper, trying to wipe it out of their life. The brooder stares at the paper, obsessing and ruminating. ("I'm too stressed! Now I'm stressed about that!) On the other hand, someone who is emotionally agile picks up the paper, turns it over and considers what the emotion means and what to do next.

Mastering this skill isn't just a happiness hack. It gives us the strength to face challenging issues head-on. Otherwise, David says, "you don't have the skills to have the tough conversation, or to think, 'Gee, is this relationship really working for me?'"

It might even be the secret to building happier, better work cultures too. David recalls working with a CEO of a multinational corporation who told her, "We want to innovate, and we want to be sustainable, and we want to be creative." Her response? "You don't get collaboration unless you are open to conflict and the idea that people may not agree with you."

It also takes emotional courage to have much-needed difficult conversations in the world at large—around systemic racism, #MeToo, and other critical issues. "It takes courage as a society for us to face these difficult emotions," David says, "but only in doing that are we able to be more resilient and intentional individuals and able to be more resilient and capable in our society."

Think of it this way, she adds: "Tough emotions are part of life. You don't get to have a meaningful career, you don't get to raise a family, and you don't get to leave the world a better place without stress and discomfort." ●

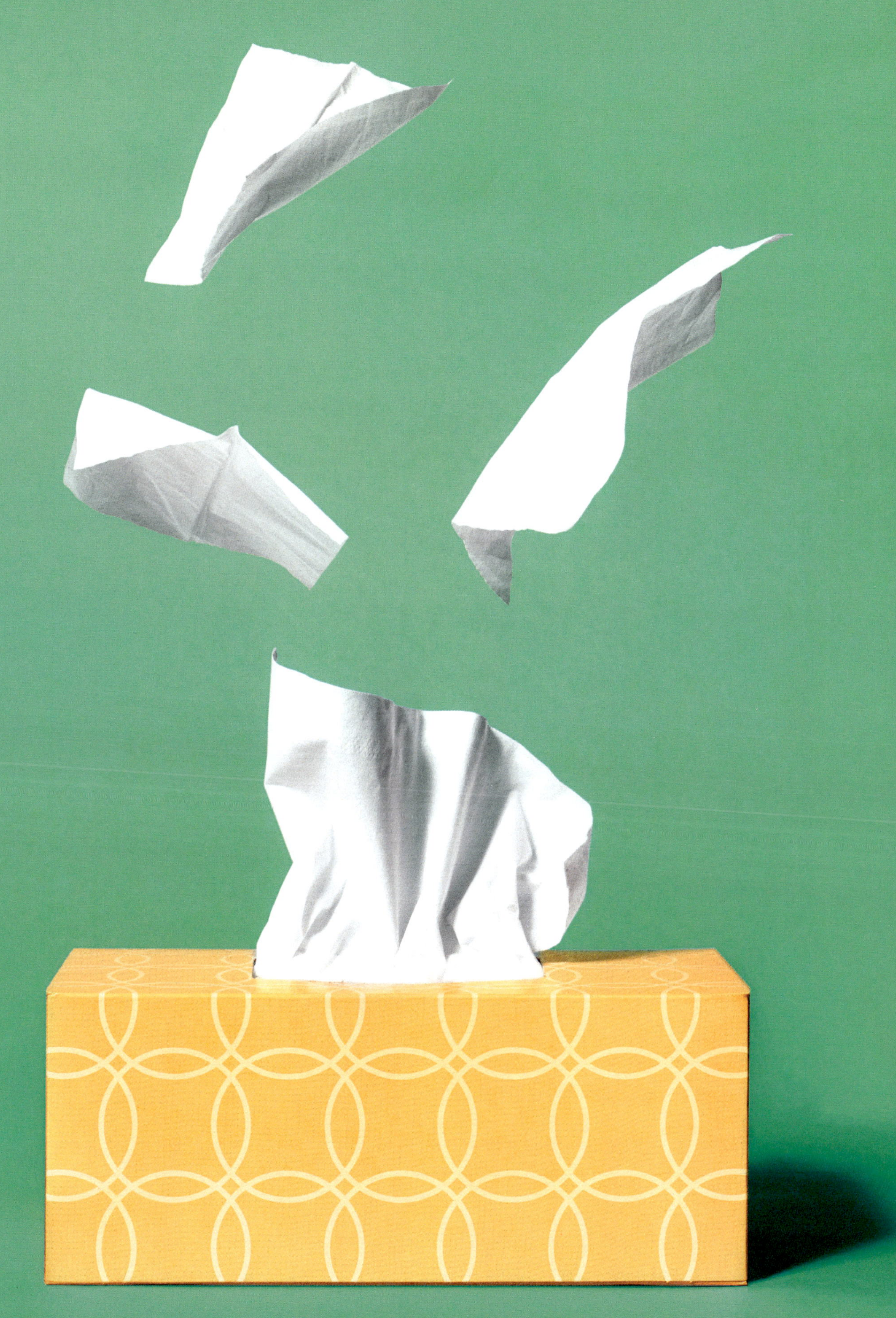

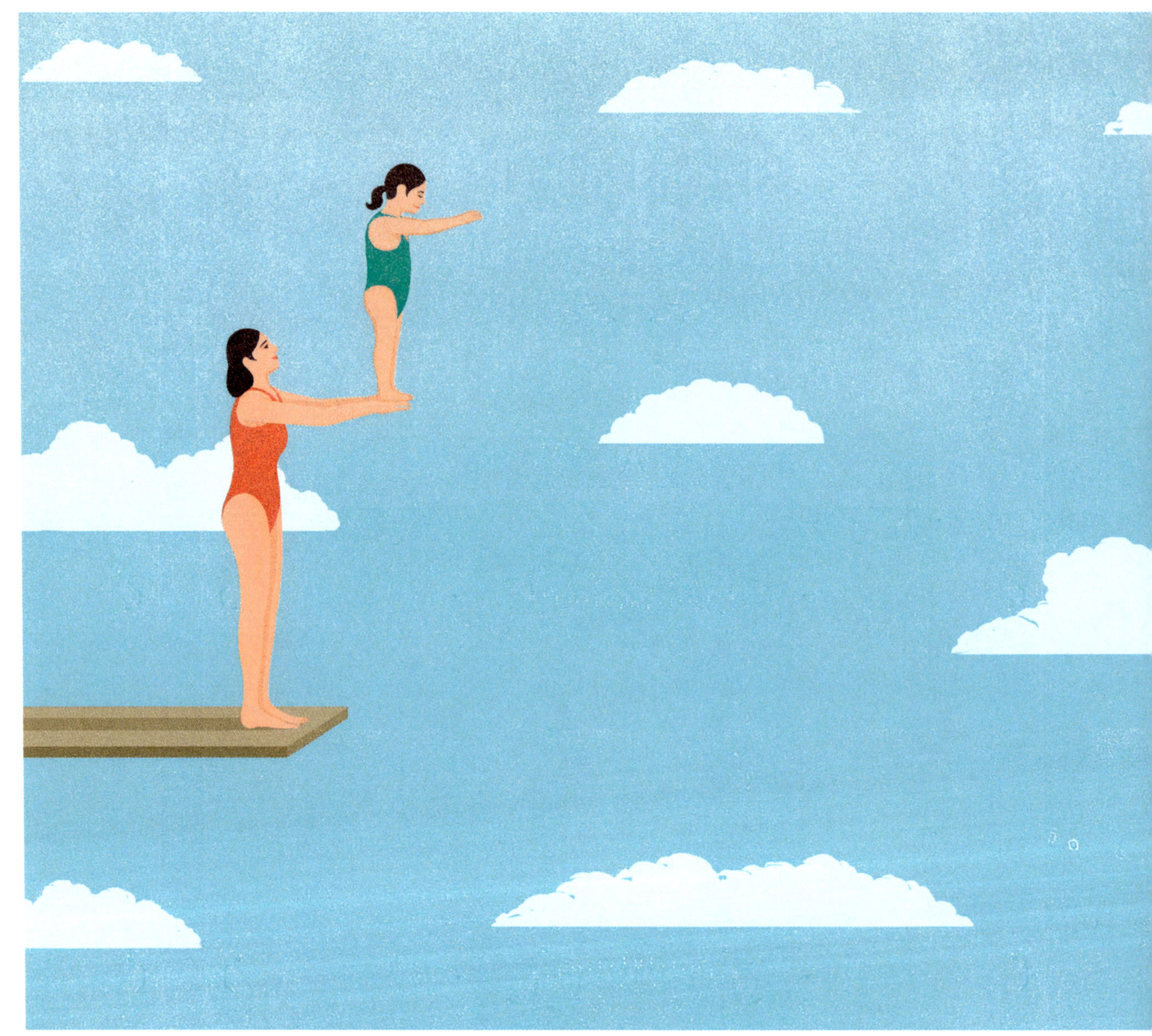

Raising a Worrier?

SIMPLE STRATEGIES TO PREPARE CHILDREN FOR THE STRESSORS LIFE WILL INEVITABLY SEND THEIR WAY—SO THEY KNOW THEY CAN COPE WITH ANYTHING.

By Juli Fraga, PsyD

FROM THE MORNING your baby cries when you leave for the first time to the day your teen comes home panicking about a bad grade, seeing your kids worry cuts like a knife. We want to protect them from suffering, but of course worrying is a normal part of childhood, adolescence, and, well, life itself. Teaching our children healthy ways to cope with the things that stress them can bolster their emotional well-being for life and prevent their worries from spiraling into something more serious, such as an anxiety disorder. Here's how to prepare the children in your life for some of the most common worries they may face, and give them the skills to cope if their fears come true.

INFANTS AND TODDLERS

The Issue: Separation Anxiety

HELP THEM PREPARE: "Separation anxiety typically begins around 10 months old and can last to about age 3 and sometimes even longer," says Nina Kaiser, PhD, a child psychologist in San Francisco. One way to help prepare little ones for goodbyes is to read a story like Anna Dewdney's *Llama Llama Misses Mama* together. "Reading books about transitions like the first day of school normalizes the experience and reassures kids that everything will turn out OK," says Kaiser. It's also smart to visit the childcare facility or school with your infants or toddlers before the first day, says Kaiser. Showing them what to expect can help them feel safer when the big day comes.

HELP THEM COPE: Children who handle separation anxiety best learn what to expect over time. Saying things like "Grown-ups always come back" when you leave and telling your child what time you will return help establish a predictable routine. Setting up a goodbye ritual by singing a song and taking your child's favorite stuffed animal to daycare can also help soothe sadness, says Kaiser. Most important, keep your own worries under wraps. "Parents' behavior shows kids whether there's something to worry about," says Kaiser. Drawing out the goodbye or becoming upset can make children's worries grow, but talking to them calmly conveys that everything is going to be fine.

The Issue: Nightmares

HELP THEM PREPARE: "Toddlers as young as 18 months old can have nightmares," says Angelique Millette, PhD, a pediatric sleep consultant with offices in Austin, Texas, and San Francisco. Nightmares can make it feel scary to go to bed the next night and even lead to fear of the dark. Though occasional bad dreams may be inevitable, Millette says that poor sleep quality can make nightmares worse. To get ahead of these overnight woes, she recommends creating a healthy sleep routine for your child. "Sticking to the same bedtime each night, using a low-watt night-light, and reading a calming story before bedtime can help kids feel safe and secure, which helps them sleep better at night," says Millette. If they're sleeping badly, make sure it isn't because they're overtired: Toddlers need about 10 to 12 hours each night and a 1½- to 2-hour nap.

HELP THEM COPE: Despite your best efforts, nightmares may still happen. And "some children become so worried about nightmares that they protest going to sleep," says Millette. With younger toddlers, she recommends leaving a light on in the hallway and sitting with them when they're distressed. Comforting statements like "You had a scary dream, but you're safe" and "Your body is good at sleeping" can also be calming. Toddlers may have difficulty naming their fears, but having them draw a picture or helping them write a story about the experience can assist them in expressing their emotions, which feels empowering.

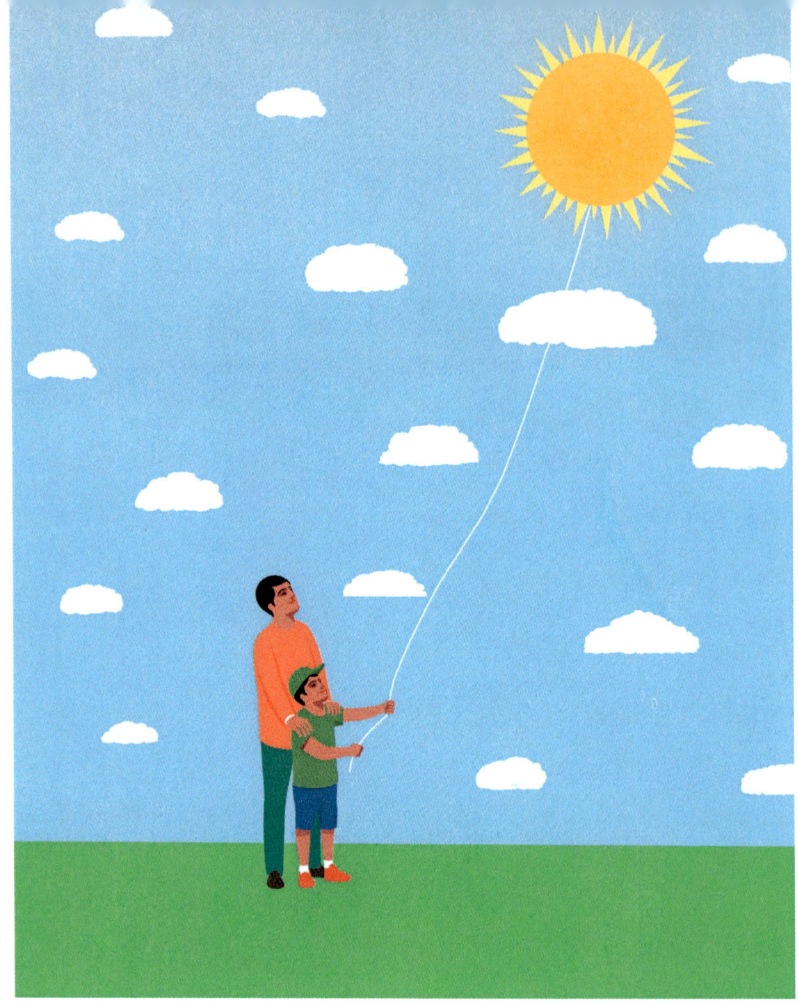

BIG KIDS

The Issue: Fear of Death

HELP THEM PREPARE: Around age 7 or earlier, many children ask their parents, "What happens after we die?" According to grief therapist Claire Bidwell Smith, the author of *Anxiety: the Missing Stage of Grief,* "When kids ask this question, it's important to welcome their curiosity and answer honestly." Smith recommends asking, "What do you think happens?" If your child asks whether people or animals go to heaven, answer honestly based on your family's beliefs. If your family doesn't believe in the afterlife, it's OK to be upfront. "Talking about life spans of other species can help," says Smith, so the death of a pet isn't completely unexpected. When death isn't a taboo topic, it can seem less scary.

HELP THEM COPE: "Kids' worries about death may grow once they realize that their parents can't protect them from everything," says Abigail Marks, PhD, a clinical psychologist in San Francisco who specializes in grief. Concerns about dying can also become magnified after losing a beloved pet or a family member. Talk openly about their fears. "See if you can find out more about their specific concerns and show that you take their feelings seriously," advises Marks. No one has the answers to all of life's existential questions, but Marks says that when kids feel reassured and understood, anxiety can begin to shrink.

The Issue: Tragedies and Disasters

HELP THEM PREPARE: Whether it's the possibility of a school shooting or a natural disaster like a hurricane, worries about tragedies can rattle a kid's sense of safety. "Parents can keep these worries at bay by being mindful about how their children are exposed to the news and to information shared online," says Kaiser. Parents also often have (legitimate) worries about this one, so lean into your support system to talk about your fears, see a therapist, or find a parents' group to join. "Parents' emotional reactions inform kids' thoughts, feelings, and behavior. If parents are anxious, kids worry more too," says Kaiser.

HELP THEM COPE: The toughest time is the immediate aftermath of a tragedy. "Facts are your friends," says Sheryl Ziegler, PsyD, a child psychologist in Denver and the author of *Mommy Burnout.* "Offer grounding statements like 'Tragedies do happen, but it's unlikely there will be one at your school,'" recommends Ziegler. If your child still seems worried, review your school's safety plan. As you discuss the details, point out teachers and staffers who monitor kids' safety every day. Look at the weather forecast together and calmly review safety and evacuation procedures.

TWEENS AND TEENS

The Issue: Friendship and Social Media

HELP THEM PREPARE: "Drama almost always comes with the territory in the social lives of teens," says Lisa Damour, PhD, a clinical psychologist and the author of *Under Pressure: Confronting the Epidemic of Stress and Anxiety in Girls.* Letting adolescents know that friendships don't exist without tension reassures them that social challenges are normal and eases their fears of peer rejection. Teens may bristle when parents give advice, but sharing that you've faced similar conflicts with friends can validate their emotions.

HELP THEM COPE: Situations like not getting invited to a party and later learning about it on Instagram can be crushing for many adolescents. "If your teen is worried about being left out in real life or on social media, empathize with their feelings. Let them know that it's hard to have that much information about what they're missing," says Damour. Noting some reasons why people may limit their guest lists can help: Maybe the party space was small, or their parents made them invite family friends. And remind your teen that hanging out with a mix of people is a normal part of social life. She can and should too.

The Issue: College Admissions

HELP THEM PREPARE: "Teaching kids how to take responsibility for their schoolwork can help them prepare for the stress of college preparation," says Jean McPhee, PhD, a clinical psychologist based in Northern California who specializes in treating learning problems and stress in students. And parents don't need to wait until their teens are in high school to instill these helpful habits. "Instead of focusing on what kids aren't doing, parents can get a step ahead of the commotion by praising them for positive behavior, like completing homework on time," says McPhee. Saying things like "I notice you got your report written—great job" reinforces the development of good time-management skills and sturdy study habits, she says.

HELP THEM COPE: Working with your teens to establish a self-care routine helps buffer them from college-prep anxiety: Stress-management techniques like exercise and healthy eating can go a long way to keep them on an even keel. And, as ever, keep your own stress about their college plans in check too. "Worried parents may react by saying something like 'You're never going to get your essays completed,' which can feed a kid's doomsday thinking," McPhee says. ●

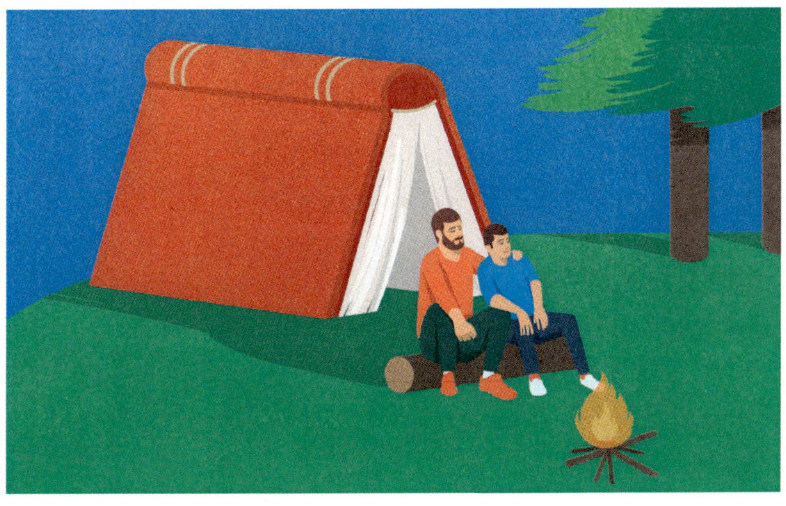

WHEN SHOULD YOU WORRY ABOUT THEIR WORRYING?

Discerning between normal kid fears and an anxiety disorder isn't always easy. The American Psychological Association notes that these signs could indicate that your child may need to see a mental-health professional:

- Health complaints: symptoms such as headaches, stomachaches, and insomnia.
- Avoidance: refusing social invites, staying home from school, or skipping sports or other activities.
- Behavioral changes: isolating themselves from friends and family members for extended periods.

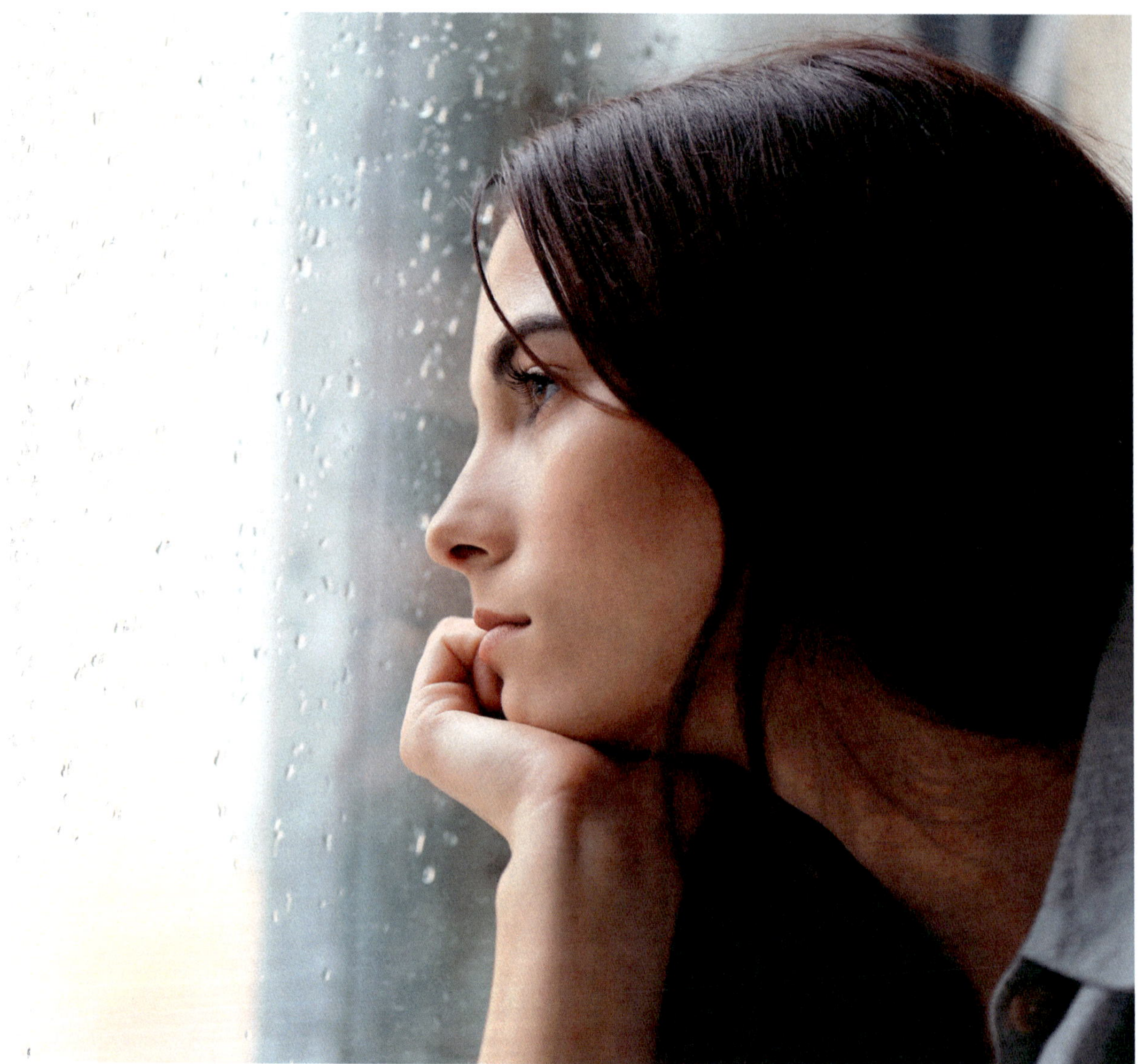

Should You Let Go of That Grudge?

A FAMILY FEUD. A COLD WAR WITH A NEIGHBOR. A WORKPLACE INJUSTICE. IT MIGHT FEEL RIGHT TO HOLD ON TO A SENSE OF BEING WRONGED—BUT YOU MAY END UP ONLY PUNISHING YOURSELF.

By Melanie Mannarino

SEARCH YOUR HEART for a minute: Are you holding any grudges? Maybe your blood still boils whenever you remember getting laid off five years ago. Or perhaps you're still seething about that comment your sister made last month. Or you still can't move past how Grandma (RIP) favored your cousin when you were kids. (Full disclosure: That last example is all mine. It took me decades to get over my grandmother comparing my "beautiful" cousin to child actress Brooke Shields. I got compared to exactly nobody.)

It's perfectly natural to bear grudges of all sizes—against a relative who showed favoritism, against a partner who cheated on you, and worse. And it's hard for most of us to let them go, says sociologist Christine Carter, PhD, the author of *The Sweet Spot: How to Accomplish More by Doing Less.* "For many people, it's easy to hang on to resentment," she says. When we've been wronged, it feels validating to think of ourselves as a blameless, oppressed victim. But playing that role makes it hard to move on, because it makes you powerless—you can't have it both ways, says Carter.

It took Mina, a 39-year-old payroll executive and mother of two, years to realize she couldn't fully move forward with her life as long as she was holding a grudge against her controlling father. "My father had anger issues and old-world views about a woman's role. When I was a teenager, we had a huge fight, and he threatened me with physical violence," she says. She cut off contact with him for more than five years. "I wished all kinds of evil on him. But after a while, I had accomplished so much on my own and was starting to think, 'I can't go on to new adventures and positive experiences if I still have this anger.'"

Harboring resentment toward someone who has insulted, demeaned, cheated on, or otherwise hurt you doesn't empower you. It can actively cause you harm, both physically and emotionally. Repeatedly recalling the slight (yes, it can definitely feel much larger than "slight") is called ruminating, says Everett Worthington, PhD, a professor emeritus of psychology at Virginia Commonwealth University, who has spent his career studying forgiveness. "Research shows that when people keep ruminating, it increases the base level of the stress hormone cortisol in their bloodstream," he says. "That in turn can shrink the brain and also impact the immune system, cardiovascular system, GI system, sex drive—there are a lot of costs."

Research bears out the health benefits of forgiveness. In a study of young adults, higher levels of forgiveness were connected to fewer physical issues, like sleep problems, digestive trouble, and headaches, as well as fewer feelings of worthlessness, hopelessness, anxiety, and depression.

If your lingering anger toward the neighbors who wronged you ends up compromising your health, "the effects of the injustice are worse than the injustice itself," says Robert Enright, PhD, a professor of educational psychology at the University of Wisconsin–Madison. It's like you've been hurt twice, and that's not really what you want, right?

What you want (presumably) is to move on and feel good about yourself and the world while making sure the offense doesn't happen again. The only way to get there is through forgiveness. "Resentment is a slow, happiness-stealing poison," says Enright. "And forgiveness is like medicine."

By Enright's definition, forgiveness is being good to those who are not good to you. Difficult, yes, but the payoff is worth it. "Think of yourself as someone who has the power to create the life you want to create," says Carter. "Showing mercy to the people who wrong us is a little-known secret to happiness."

Mina found happiness in her 20s while visiting friends over Easter break. "I woke up in Italy, and the bells were ringing at the nearby church, and the sky was filled with light pink and purple," she recalls. "I was happy in that moment, appreciative of my friends, and thankful I was living the exact way I wanted to live. I silently said to my father, 'I forgive you. I love you! I thank you for my life. I wish you well and hope you are all right.' That was it. I released my anger and hatred for him that morning."

Ready to release your own hurt? Set aside everything you think you know about holding grudges and follow these expert guidelines for letting them go and lightening your emotional load.

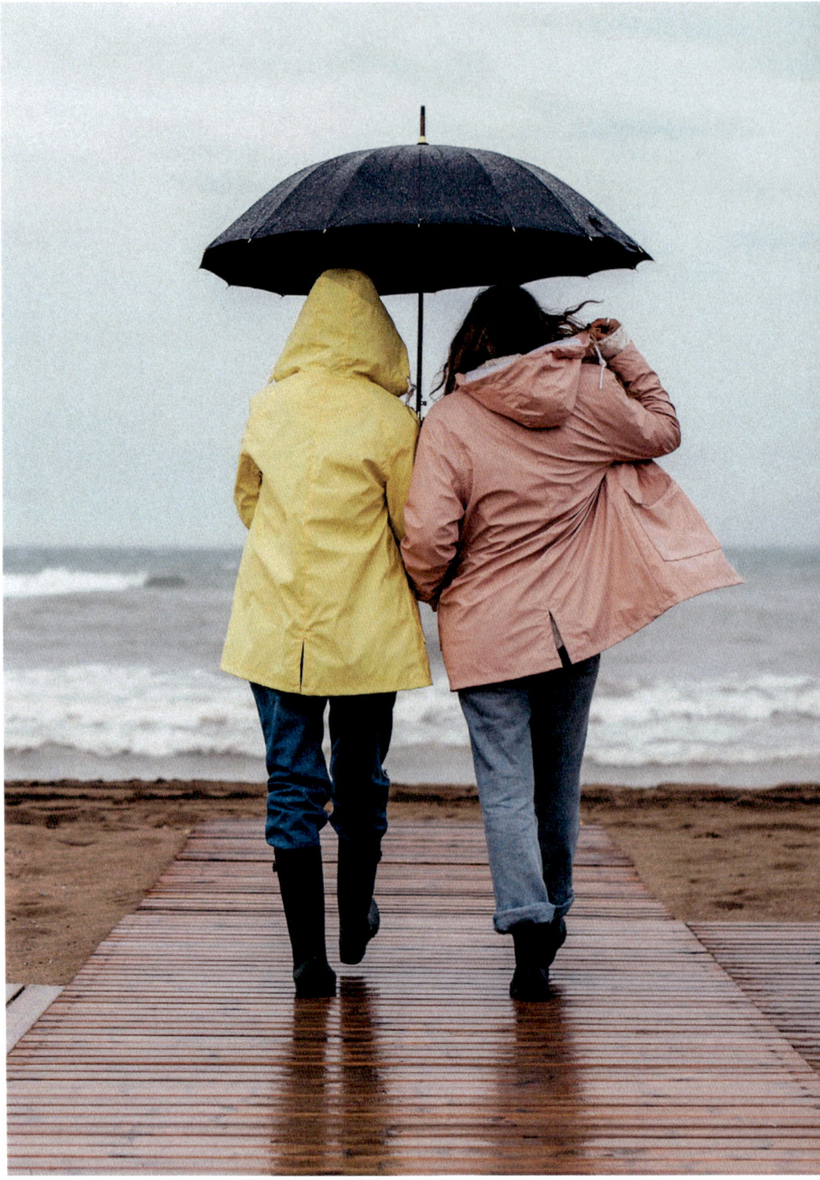

Consider what is good for you

"In holding a grudge, there's a sense of strength and righteousness in the short term," notes Enright. "You're saying, 'You can't do this to me.' The quest for justice seems right. But it does not cure the resentment." It's not about whether the offender deserves forgiveness. "You deserve it," says Enright, "because you are the one who is hurt. You deserve to live a life free of that gnawing and discontent."

See the other person through new eyes

It may feel like the offender's actions were meant to hurt you—and sometimes that's true. But Enright encourages everyone to view these incidents from a different perspective. "Don't define the person by the words or action that hurt you," he says. "That is not all the person is. Try to see them more broadly, in terms of their humanity and when they might have done good. You'll see the weaknesses they have never overcome—that is a tragedy for them, making them and others miserable. When people are consistently mean to us, especially in families, there is likely something deeper going on. The offer of forgiveness is healing for both of you. You don't have to excuse them, but say, 'Here's a person who could be living a fuller life but isn't.'"

It's OK to recall the hurt, adds Worthington. But when doing so, replace the negative emotions with more positive ones of empathy or sympathy for the offender.

Don't wait for someone to "earn" your forgiveness. It's an altruistic gift, says Worthington. "People don't deserve forgiveness. They don't earn it. We simply give it."

Carter's advice: Do it sooner rather than later. "A lot of people hold grudges because they are waiting for an apology," she says. "They think, 'I'll forgive her, but she hasn't asked me yet.' But that's not the way the world works. Most people won't apologize in a way that is satisfying—in our culture we aren't really taught how to do it. So if we want to be happy and heal ourselves when we've been hurt, we must forgive whether or not we are asked for forgiveness."

Anna, a 35-year-old writer and mom of one, spent years nursing a grudge against a teacher who cut her from show choir in seventh grade—even after they both moved on to the high school. "For the first two years of high school, I would not speak to her or look her in the eye," she admits. "But the first day of junior year, I was like, 'This is silly. I don't care.' So that day, I smiled at her. After that, I really enjoyed her class—and we are still in touch, nearly 20 years later. I'm glad for both of us that I gave her a second chance. Smiling at her was way less emotionally taxing than holding all that negative energy."

Separate forgiveness from reconciliation

By forgiving someone, you are not validating their behavior, the experts agree. This is especially important to remember in more serious situations, including cases of abuse, legal strife, or marital infidelity. Reconciliation is mutual; forgiveness is not. Even if you've suffered a huge injustice, says Enright, "you can offer the gift of goodness to the other person, knowing they made a mistake—whether or not they understand what they've done, are sorry for it, or try to make reparations."

When people do not forgive, says Enright, they tend to pass their resentment on to others. "In a family, the children inherit the anger," he says. "The innocent ones inherit the resentment that shouldn't be theirs. They grow up with an anger, and if they enter into a marital union, they bring that anger into the new relationship."

Forgive freely, but don't necessarily forget

Instead, reframe the relationship. Say you haven't spoken with your sister in 15 years, and lately you've been thinking of burying your grudge. Go ahead—but know that you have a right to redefine the relationship. You can forgive her parenting criticism and still choose not to vacation with her anymore. "A lot of times, we hold on to grudges to give ourselves permission to not bridge a divide," says Carter. "But you don't need the grudge to create safety for yourself. Forgive her, but keep the boundary: If you know your sister is always going to hurt you, I wouldn't recommend spending Christmas at her house. Don't expose yourself to future harm."

After forgiving her father, Mina didn't renew their relationship. "I know that in the end, I made the right decision for me and for him," she says. "I thought we might say one last goodbye before he died. But it's OK—I've let him go and all the baggage that came with him."

Find the lesson in the offense

In her book *How to Hold a Grudge*, author Sophie Hannah explores the positive side of grudges—namely, the things they can teach you about how you want to live your life and interact with others. What stays with you, says Hannah, is the story you choose to remember about an incident that made you feel wronged or hurt. "The grudge becomes a story you can use to improve your life and guide you and provide inspiration," she explains. "When you form a grudge against someone for bad behavior, it inspires you to behave in the opposite way." In time, you may even become grateful for the opportunity to avoid similar bad behavior and for the example of how not to treat others.

Confront the offender only if it will change things

"If you think someone will deny their actions and criticize you for being overly sensitive, it's better to show you forgive than to proclaim it," says Enright. "Return a phone call or text, smile in the office hallway, pay them a visit—be good to them in a genuine sense. They will understand." If reconciliation does seem possible, he says, you can sit down with the person and tell them, "You hurt me, and I'd like for us to avoid having that happen again."

Know that it's never too late—really

"You can even forgive someone who is deceased," notes Enright. "You can take an inventory of the injustices of your life, from your first-grade teacher up to your boss yesterday, and practice forgiving everybody so they don't 'win' twice. If you hold on to it, they win again. Forgive them, and it takes away their power." ●

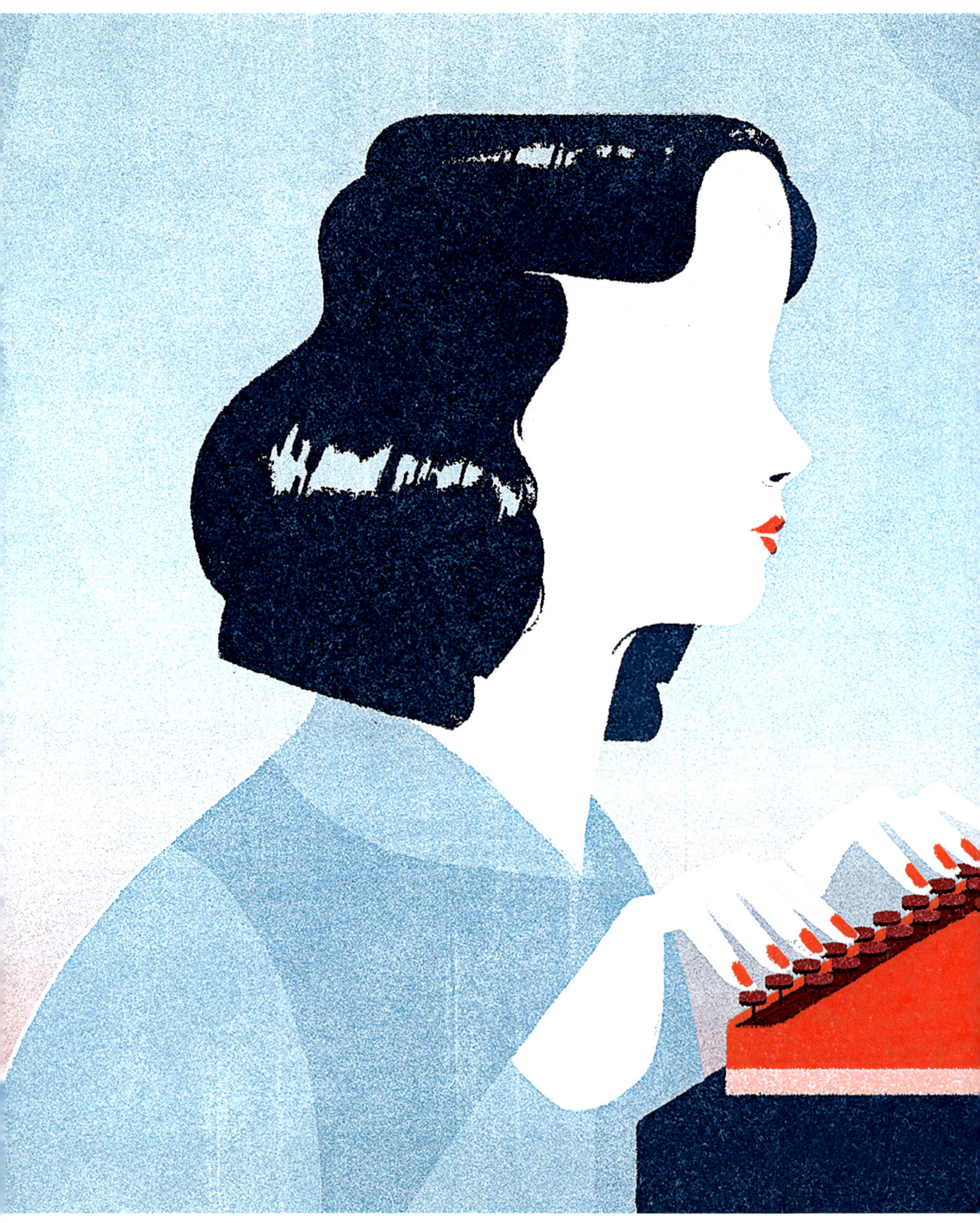

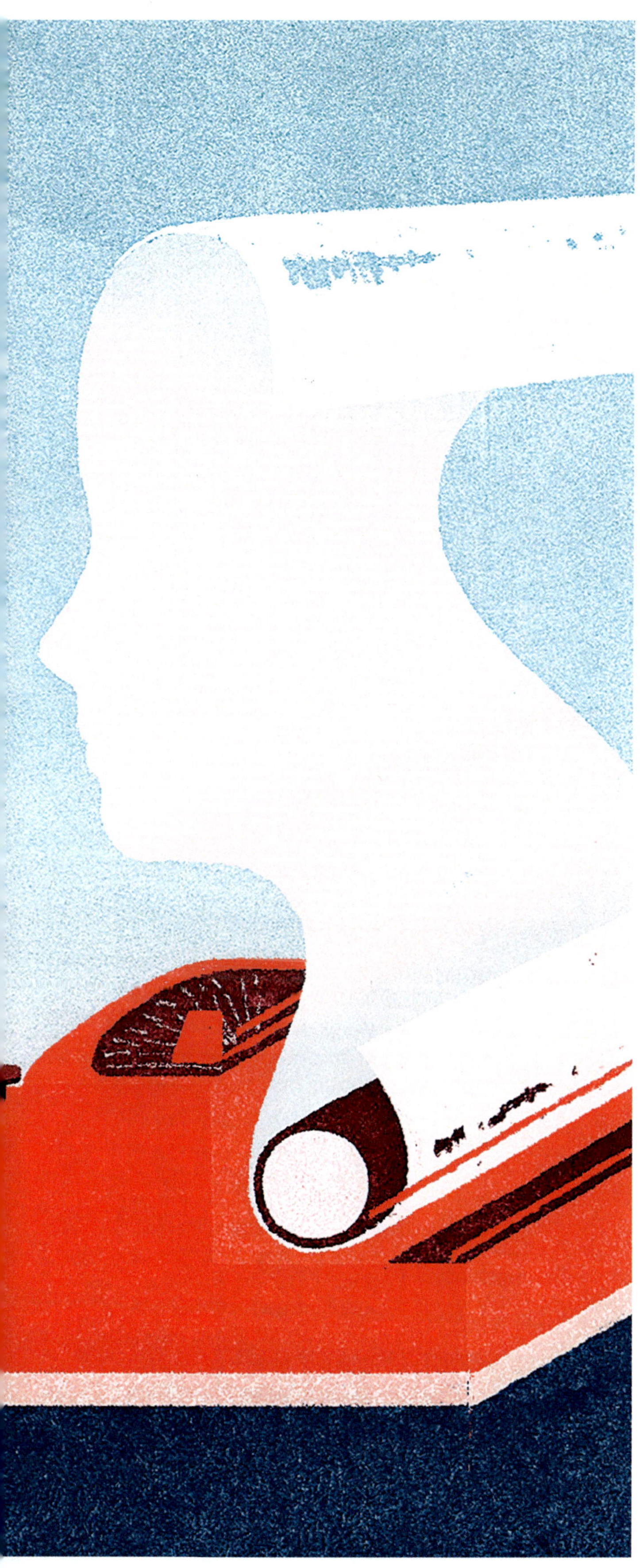

The Power of Your Story

WE NATURALLY THINK OF OUR LIVES AS STORIES. CHANGING THE WAY YOU TELL YOURS CAN HELP YOU HANDLE WHATEVER PLOT TWISTS COME YOUR WAY.

By Jennifer King Lindley

HUMANS ARE transfixed by stories. We freeze—popcorn handful in midair—when the movie hero finally comes face-to-face with the villain. We stay up way too late to see how a potboiler ends even though we're too grown-up to hide a flashlight under the covers. We get lost in the experiences of strangers through podcasts like *The Moth* and *StoryCorps* and of our friends via Instagram and Snapchat.

Stories are how we naturally conceive of our own lives as well. "Our lives are so complex that we need some way to make sense of them," says Jonathan Adler, PhD, a professor of psychology at Olin College of Engineering in Needham, Massachusetts. "When we construct a narrative, it allows us to hold on to the important parts, filter out the trivial, and find a meaningful pattern in it all."

Day-to-day life is a mash-up, after all: What you had for breakfast. The traffic jam. The birth of a child. Like an editor, our brains pull out significant conflicts, important characters, and turning points to shape our sense of who we are. You might share with a new friend your "journey" with an eating disorder, your "battle" with cancer. We're living through events while also interpreting them as we go along, says Adler. "You are both the main character and the narrator of your life," he says. "You may not have control over all your circumstances, but you can choose how to tell the story."

The problem, say experts: You're not the most reliable narrator. You might give yourself the most deflating interpretation of your circumstances. ("I got downsized: Decades of work have added up to nothing!") Or you lose the plot entirely when life throws an unexpected twist. ("How can I be struggling to get pregnant? I am meant to be a mom!") Then you go around in circles instead of moving forward. To study how we create our personal stories, researchers at Northwestern University have interviewed hundreds of people to elicit their life narratives. Their findings: Those who tend to weave "contamination stories," in which key points in life are described as tainted ("The promotion was my career goal, but now I'm stressed by the responsibility"), measure lower on levels of well-being than those who naturally tell "redemption stories" that emphasize the silver lining. ("Our bankruptcy was hard, but it brought our family closer")

It all may sound a bit too Joseph Campbell. But as this emerging field of "narrative psychology" grows, researchers and therapists are finding practical, do-right-now ways you can tweak your own inner stories. Such edits can help you become more resilient, have better relationships, and—happily ever after!—make better decisions.

1

Give yourself a more positive "story prompt"

In one influential study, Tim Wilson, PhD, a professor of psychology at the University of Virginia in Charlottesville, gathered first-year college students who were floundering academically. "Many were telling themselves pessimistic stories, like 'College is a harder place than I thought. Maybe I don't belong here,'" says Wilson, the author of *Redirect: Changing the Stories We Live By*. "If that's your story, it can really spiral downward. You think it's hopeless, so you don't try."

To get them out of this self-defeating mindset, researchers showed some of the students videotapes of older students who shared that they too had struggled at first, but once they learned the ropes, their grades climbed. Students who were exposed to this brief, one-time intervention got better grades and were more likely to stay in college than those who weren't exposed to it. "Perhaps this new prompt made them think, 'Maybe my negative story wasn't right. Maybe I just need new study skills,'" says Wilson. The mental revise spurred them to action.

You can try this kind of story edit yourself. Totally lost it with your kids after the third Popsicle accident of the day? Instead of thinking, "I'm a terrible mother for making my kids cry," try a more charitable interpretation: "Parenting little kids is a tough job for everyone." Now, who wants to play with the hose!

TRY IT: If you've had a setback, try giving your current predicament a title, suggests Schneiderman, like "1,000 Résumés: Adventures in Unemployment." Thinking of your life in chapters helps you realize your hardships likely have a finite beginning and end, so they feel less overwhelming. "This is just one twist in the long story of your life."

2

View difficult people as characters meant to teach you something

Not many enduring classics have this plotline: Everyone got along great! We grabbed lattes, did some shopping, and went home happy! Instead, the most treasured tales have antagonists—enemies our hero must use his inner strength to overcome. Where would Harry Potter be without Voldemort?

Rather than just steaming away, think of your difficult in-law or unreasonable boss as an antagonist in your story, suggests Kim Schneiderman, a licensed clinical social worker, a psychotherapist in New York

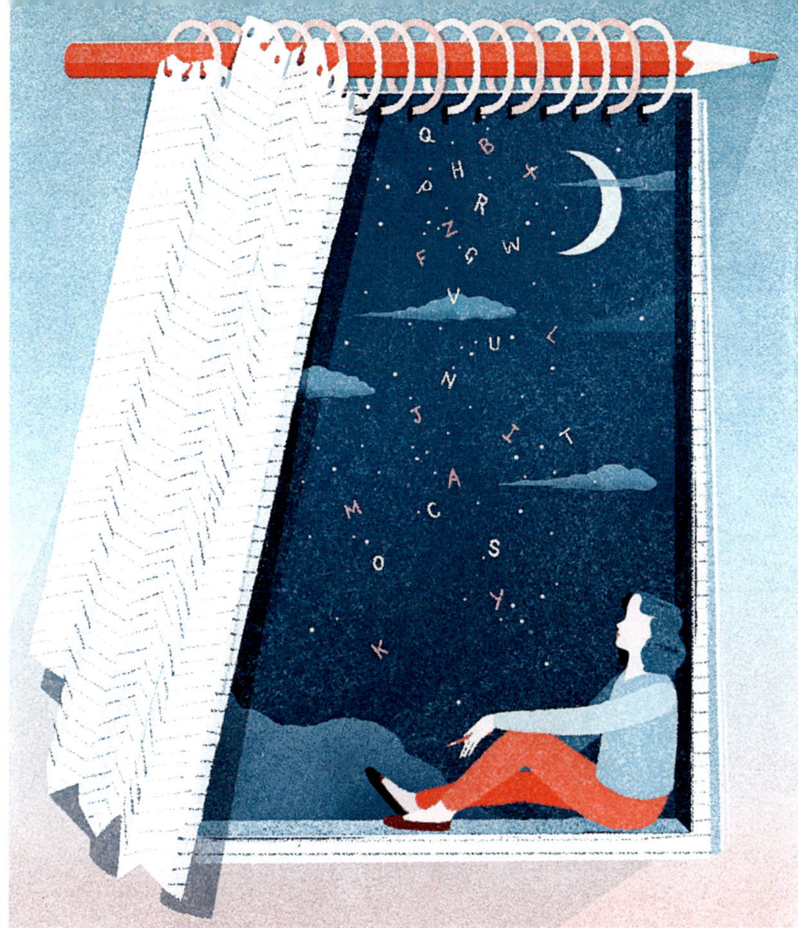

TRY IT: Hash out relationship conflicts in writing. In a study published in the journal *Psychological Science*, researchers asked couples to write about a minor conflict in their marriage (say, dirty dishes left all over) for seven minutes at a time every few months for one year. The twist: They had to adopt the perspective of a third person who had everyone's best interests at heart (in other words, channel a marriage counselor). Taking this fair-minded approach helped defuse everyday clashes and bolster marital satisfaction.

City and the author of *Step Out of Your Story: Writing Exercises to Reframe and Transform Your Life*. "Just like good fiction, life is about character development," she says. "These people push you to discover your strengths and your resources by presenting you with challenges. Ask yourself, 'What are they here to teach me?'"

To gird yourself for battle (e.g., Thanksgiving dinner with your overbearing mother-in-law), imagine yourself as the hero in a novel. "Ask yourself, 'What do I hope the main character would do in these circumstances? What would I root for the outcome to be? How might she grow from this experience?'" says Schneiderman. She suggests you even sketch out the scene in writing using the third-person voice. Be as literal or as imaginative as you like. You don't have to be Shakespeare here: Simple sentences are fine. ("Jen took a deep breath and squared her shoulders. Leveling a cool glance at the older woman, she at last said out loud what she had been thinking for years: 'Thank you for the parenting advice. But I do things differently.'")

You are not trying to script the encounter in advance, she says. "Instead, the idea is to gain some distance and recognize you have control over how you react to conflicts. This exercise kicks you out of victim mode and lets you see these kinds of small, daily challenges as a way to grow." That type of attitude shift can make you feel—and therefore act—more empowered in real life.

3

Observe yourself with some distance, as if you were a character in a book

We often feel paralyzed when facing a big decision—a career move, a breakup. Yet we have no trouble doling out brilliant advice to a friend in the same situation. Adopting a narrator's fly-on-the-wall stance can cool your emotions and let you approach your problems with the same wise detachment, says Ethan Kross, PhD, a professor of psychology at the University of Michigan in Ann Arbor.

In one of his studies, subjects were given five minutes to prepare a speech—a classic stress inducer. He asked one group to talk to themselves using "I" words. ("OMG! What if I faint dead away?!") Members of another group were told to refer to themselves as they would another person. ("Jen just needs to take a deep breath and smile.") The result: Subjects who adopted the third-person perspective were calmer and more confident and performed better than the "I" sayers.

You can try this whenever

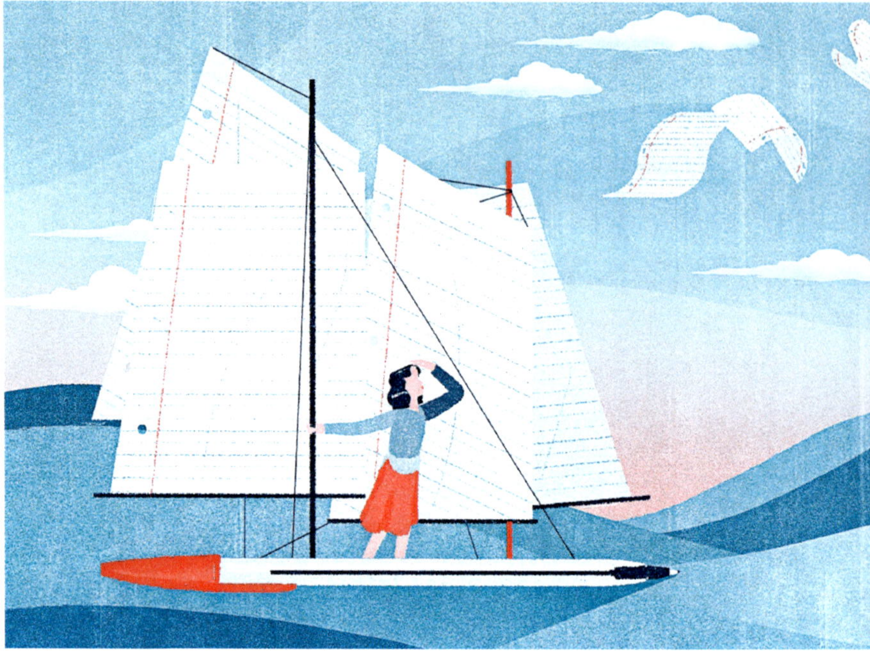

you face a stressful situation, says Kross. ("What should Jen do to make sure she doesn't blow her deadline?") Or visualize a daunting event in advance, observing yourself as if from a distance: Envision this cool customer's actions, acing the presentation and modestly accepting applause.

4

Write about a painful time to make peace with it

We want our lives to make as much sense as a well-plotted novel, with no strange turns or loose threads. That's why big setbacks are so disorienting. "No one anticipates their story will be, You graduate, get married, have kids, get cancer," says Adler. "When bad things happen, you have to find a way to fit them into the story you thought you were telling."

One well-documented way to do so is through expressive writing, a technique pioneered by James Pennebaker, a professor of psychology at the University of Texas at Austin. In studies, Pennebaker asked people to spend 15 minutes a day for four days writing about their most painful experience—a loss, an estrangement, an illness. They were asked to pour out their emotions and reflect on how the experience connected with their past, relationships, and work. Those who did this kind of writing showed a host of benefits, from less depression to fewer doctor's visits. "Writing may help you reframe the event in a more meaningful way and figure out a way to make sense of it," says Wilson.

5

Swap stories with loved ones

"We connect around stories. When we share a story, we are offering a piece of ourselves," says Anna Osborn, a marriage and family therapist in Sacramento, California. When you first met your spouse, for example, you might have stayed up till the wee hours telling tales about your past. Alas, over the years, your talk often dwindles to composing the shopping list for your next Target run. "You may be constantly interacting, but you're not connecting," says Osborn. Her prescription: sharing your stories again. Instead of asking, "How was your day?" (answer: "Fine! Yours?") ask, "What was your biggest success today? What was your biggest challenge?" These prompts make you explain the why and share the emotions behind the highs and lows. "Think about how you are supposed to act at story hour at the library. Your job is to be truly attentive," says Osborn. You can do the same with other relationships, says Osborn: a states-away sister, a dear but drifting friend. Find a distraction-free time to ask such ponderables as "What was the biggest turning point in your life?" or "What is one memory that always brings you joy?" These questions, she says, "ask us to search deep into who we really are, what makes us tick, which allows for real connection." How's that for a happy ending? ●

TRY IT: Hearing real-life stories in which relatives, past and present, faced adversity but triumphed boosts kids' resilience, according to research from the Family Narratives Project at Emory University. So share family victories. Regale your kids with tales of how Grandma and Grandpa dug their way out of bankruptcy and started the family business, or how Aunt Jodie survived a grave childhood illness and—joy!—grew up to become mom to their favorite cousins.

Life Lessons We Learn from Kids

Seeing the world through younger eyes can shift our perspective in powerful ways.

By Kimberly Truong

1. How to confront (and embrace) your fears

My daughter has been obsessed with death for most of her life, and it can get pretty intense sometimes. She doesn't know anyone who died; it's just that, when she began to understand the concept, it was really scary to her. I was always like, "Well, let's talk about death and get to the root of where your fear comes from." But what actually helped her was dressing up in her glow-in-the-dark skeleton pajamas, putting on all her glow-in-the-dark monster fingers and vampire teeth, getting in the closet, lighting herself up, and then coming out into the dark room and pretending to be Death. Embodying it didn't make her fear of death go away, but it made the intensity of it diminish.

HILLARY FRANK IS THE CREATOR OF THE PODCAST *THE LONGEST SHORTEST TIME* AND THE AUTHOR OF *WEIRD PARENTING WINS*.

2. How to relate to other people, even when they seem different

My young readers remind me how similar we all are beneath the surface—we're all human. Instead of seeing my book *American Panda* as an Asian story, young readers see it as the coming-of-age story that it is, and they see the protagonist, Mei, as the American teen she is. In some ways, Mei does have a different background from many, but everyone can relate to having conflict with loved ones, feeling like they don't measure up, or struggling with where they fit in the world. Kids aren't as quick to assign labels, and I hope we can follow their lead more.

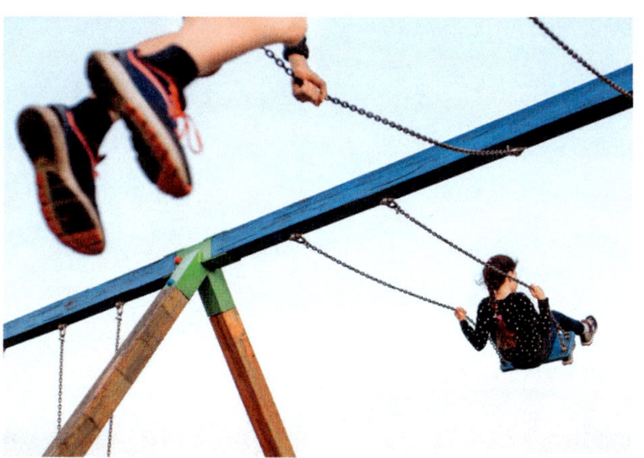

GLORIA CHAO IS THE AUTHOR OF *AMERICAN PANDA, OUR WAYWARD FATE* AND *RENT A BOYFRIEND*.

3. How to find joy in the most mundane parts of the day-to-day

I was once running errands with my daughter. I parked the car and then let her put the money in the meter. She sighed happily and said, "I just love putting money in the parking meter." And she meant it! Everything is new to her. One of the pleasures of being around young kids is borrowing some of that wonder, and allowing more space to notice the joy in things that seem mundane—even a parking meter.

EILEEN KENNEDY-MOORE, PHD, IS A CLINICAL PSYCHOLOGIST AND A COAUTHOR OF *GROWING FRIENDSHIPS: A KID'S GUIDE TO MAKING AND KEEPING FRIENDS*.

4. How to make time for bonding rituals

My 2-year-old grandson remembers the little things we do together. One of our traditions is going to the playground, and he rides on my shoulders on our way there. After we spend a bit of time cracking acorns, swinging, or kicking around leaves, he'll say he wants to go to the coffee shop and get a muffin. It's our particular ritual, and we've been doing it for over a year. Each time he's at my house for the day, he'll bring this up. I'm struck by how deeply he knows me and how he's developed a set of things he does with me that he remembers. If I'm willing to follow his lead, it demonstrates to him that I'm there for him and that our relationship is something he can count on. It's a way to build a secure attachment.

MICHAEL REICHERT, PHD, IS AN APPLIED AND RESEARCH PSYCHOLOGIST AND THE AUTHOR OF *HOW TO RAISE A BOY: THE POWER OF CONNECTION TO BUILD GOOD MEN*.

5. How not to hold back

I'm always noticing the way kids don't alter their emotions. The experience of, say, having a child nonchalantly tell you they love you, randomly throughout the day, the way a grown-up might say they enjoy coffee, can be overwhelming if you don't have kids, when you're not accustomed to trafficking in emotions so freely. I appreciate how children let themselves be so vulnerable and, unlike adults, don't try to contain their feelings. It can be really freeing not to worry what anyone else thinks.

GLYNNIS MACNICOL IS THE AUTHOR OF *NO ONE TELLS YOU THIS: A MEMOIR*.

Relearning to Drive

IN FACING A PHOBIA, ONE WRITER GETS A REFRESHER COURSE IN THE TWISTS AND TURNS OF LIFE.

By Marjorie Ingall
Photo Narrative by Holly Andres

I CONSIDER MYSELF lucky in love and unlucky in cars. When I was 12, my dad fell asleep while driving us home from a visit to Grandma's. We hit a telephone pole at 30 miles per hour. I broke my femur (the thickest bone in the human body) and had to be cut out of the car with the Jaws of Life. I had two surgeries and spent months on crutches and in physical therapy.

For a few months afterward, I was jittery in cars. But I got over it. I was young and resilient. Eventually I turned 16 and got my license. Although I was slightly anxious behind the wheel at first (I have the sense of direction of a houseplant), I became a little more comfortable each time I put the key in the ignition.

Then, when I was 18, I was slammed back to square one: As a camp counselor on a night off, I went to an ice cream parlor with four of my fellow wholesome teens. On our drive back to camp, a skunk ran across the curving country road. The driver, who had only recently gotten her license, panicked. She lost control and swerved wildly back and forth until we hit a parked milk truck. I went through the windshield and broke a shoulder blade and a finger. I crawled to someone's lawn, across broken glass, as fast as I could. Everyone in

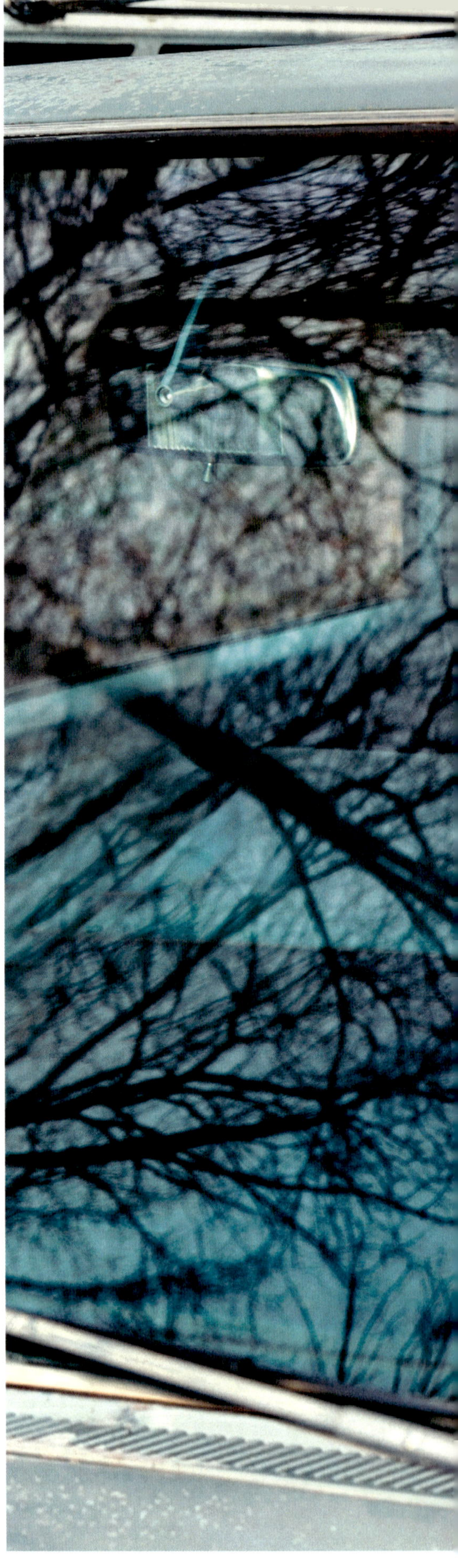

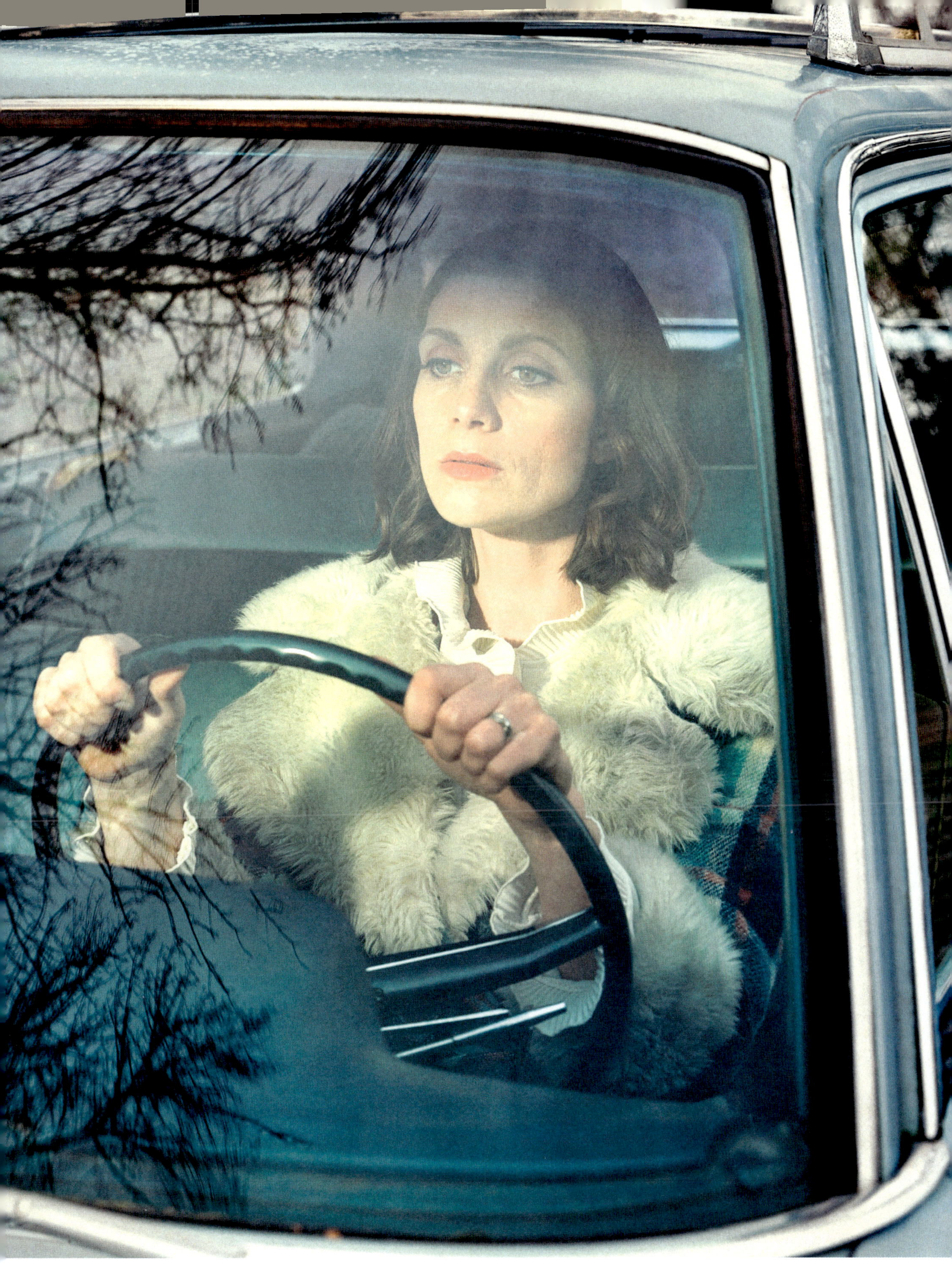

the car was injured, but no one died. Later, when we saw a picture in the newspaper of our car in the junkyard, it was so squashed and splintered, it seemed impossible that anyone had survived.

I grew up. I drove when I had to. Because I lived in New York City, there wasn't much occasion to. But I got behind the wheel when I was visiting my family in Rhode Island or traveling for work.

When I met my husband-to-be, Jonathan, I moved to San Francisco for a time. Everyone there drove very slowly and got stuck at four-way intersections smiling at one another, inching forward, stopping, smiling some more. It was annoying but predictable, and therefore manageable.

Eventually we moved back to NYC, now more than a decade ago, and had kids. Since I was hardly ever called upon to drive, my fear—always lurking in the shadows like a mugger—got worse. I turned down invitations to friends' houses if my husband couldn't drive or if I couldn't take public transportation. I passed on the crazy-cool Korean water spa in Queens unless someone could take me. My life started to feel more and more circumscribed. Being afraid to drive felt like a metaphor for passivity and dependence—and it was a huge and ever increasing source of tension between my husband and me.

Thanks, I'll walk

When Jonathan drove, I'd stare wide-eyed at the road, making reflexive squeaks and jerks. It drove him nuts. Not only did it distract him but it also made him feel that I didn't trust him behind the wheel. He sometimes felt as trapped as I did, knowing that we could never move to a place where I'd be called upon to drive.

Then, a couple of years ago, in the middle of the night, we were driving with our kids to a vacation in Steamboat Springs, Colorado. Jonathan was behind the wheel; our girls, 8 and 11 at the time, were in back. It was pitch-black and the road was deserted. Out of nowhere, right in our headlights and filling the windshield, were two giant brown bodies. Elk. I felt my skin get hot and time slow down and blood rush to my head and then the noise and a pow. All four airbags inflated. For a moment, I had no clue where I was and thought I was blind. (My past crashes had been in airbag-free cars.) The kids screamed, but I became totally calm, living the moment I'd half-expected since I was 18 years old.

The car was totaled, but we were OK. The girls sobbed to see the dead elk on the side of the road. A nice trucker offered us a lift to our hotel. It wasn't until we arrived that I saw I had a giant slash on my arm, from elbow to shoulder. I didn't want to go to the ER. I still have a scar.

I wouldn't get behind the wheel after that. Then, last summer, Jonathan and I had a fight. Like most fights, it started off being about one thing but became about others. One of those was driving. We were at my mother-in-law's house in Wisconsin, and I couldn't even storm off after the fight because I would have had to drive. I felt ridiculous and powerless, unable to even make a dramatic exit. Suddenly I became determined to face my fears, clip on the damn seat belt, and get into gear.

I couldn't even storm off after the fight, because I would have had to drive. I felt ridiculous, unable to even make a dramatic exit.

Caution: student driver

I started researching. I'd wanted to use one of those immersive virtual-reality machines—like *Grand Theft Auto* in a giant egg—but I couldn't find one anywhere nearby. What I did find was a Long Island driving school called A Woman's Way. "Phobia counseling for licensed and unlicensed drivers," the website said. The founder, Lynn S. Fuchs, had served on the Department of Motor Vehicles' advisory board for years. She'd helped rewrite the curriculum for prospective driving instructors. Her teaching methods were cited in the state DMV's driving manual. She worked with only one other instructor—a woman named Myra. (Come on, how can you not trust a Myra?) On the phone, Lynn assured me that I could learn to cope with my driving anxiety, putting me instantly at ease with her friendly Long Island accent. She scoffed at my desire to use a driving simulator.

("You need to actually do it!") I made an appointment.

The night before my first lesson, I lay awake staring at the ceiling. (I'd have counted sheep, except they'd probably have jumped into the path of a speeding SUV.) In the morning, I took a train out to a place called Valley Stream. Lynn's associate, Myra, picked me up at the station. Myra was in her 60s, with bright orange hair and a hypnotically soothing voice, plus that same reassuring motherly accent. Still, my hands were shaking. "The anticipation is the worst part," Myra promised.

As she drove to a quiet neighborhood where I could get behind the wheel, she surprised me with her use of the horn at an intersection. I grew up thinking that anyone who used a horn was rude. Myra noted placidly, "I think of the horn as a conversation." Sensing my doubt, she explained: "Your horn is your voice. It's how you express yourself. You use it when you're not sure another driver knows you're there. You're not being rude; you're saying, 'Hey, I'm here.'" This felt oddly like a feminist lesson, and I determined I was in good hands.

Myra pulled over. We sat in the car for a few minutes talking. My fear, we discovered, focused on two things: not knowing what was going to happen and not being in control of a situation. But, Myra noted, when you're driving, you are in control—you're more in control than you are as a passenger. She had a point.

"Drive," she said

It was time to switch seats. I felt as if I were swallowing a giant rock as I walked around the car, opened the driver's-side door, and slipped inside. "Adjust the seat," Myra prodded. She showed me that she had her own brake and could stop the car if I got in trouble. She could grab the wheel if I froze or panicked. And she revealed a secret weapon: The student-driving car was equipped with an oversize rearview mirror. It was as big as a loaf of bread! I looked into it and heard angels singing. I could see so much more. Noting my excitement, Myra said, "You get one of these when we're done! Anyone can buy one!" It snaps right onto the regular mirror. "People may laugh," she continued, "but when they see it in action, they always want one."

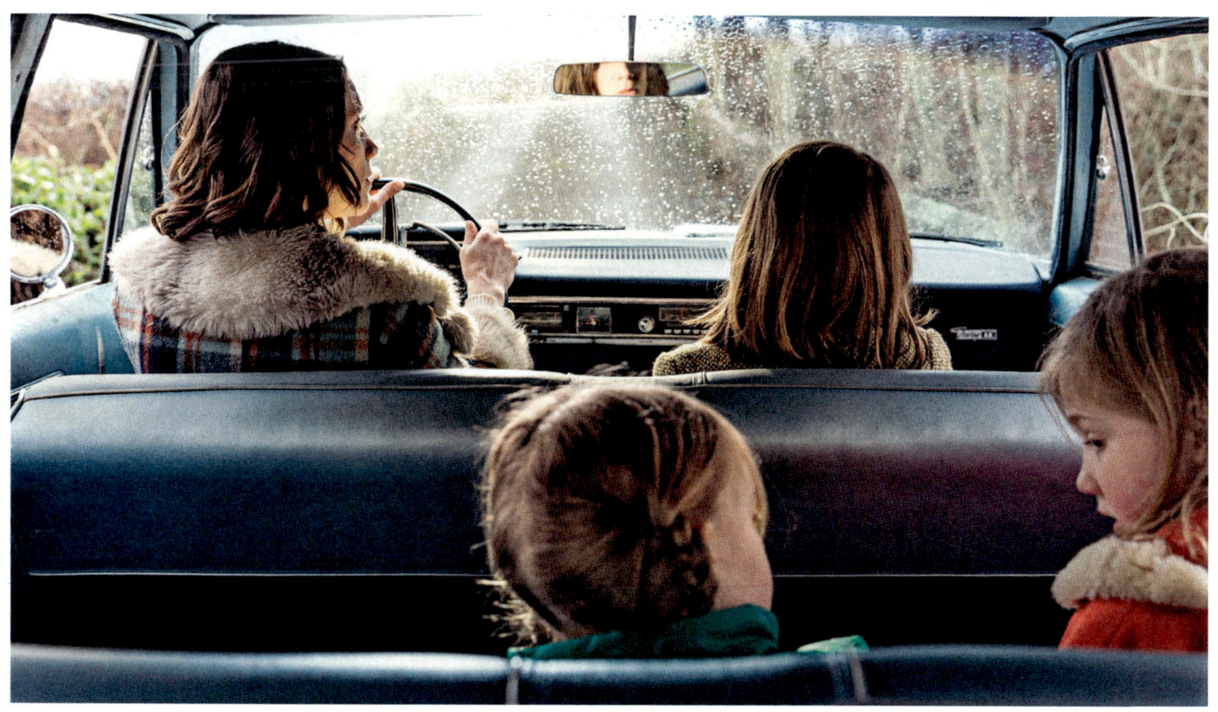

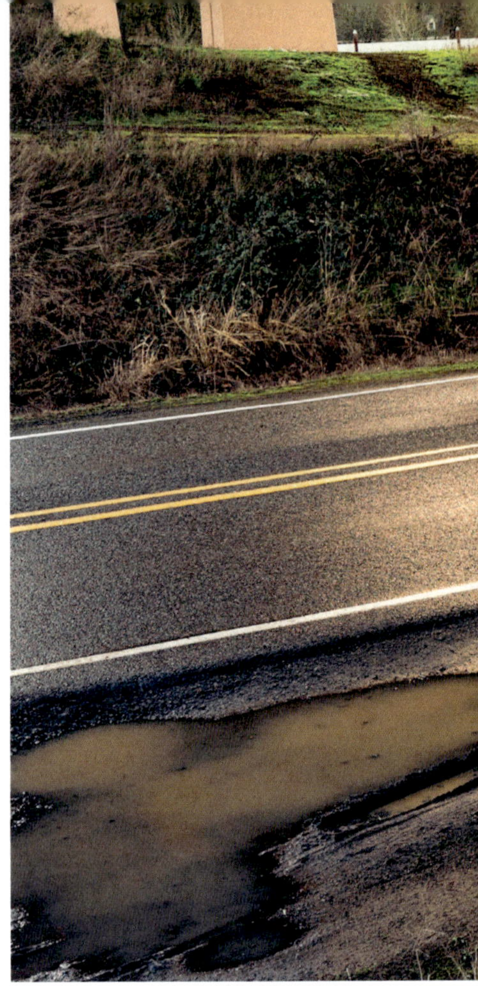

When you're attuned to your environment and open to possibility, you can be ready for adventure and more attentive to life's quirky moments. The fear of driving itself was what I'd been fearing, to lousily paraphrase FDR.

We went through the pre-driving protocols: seat belt, mirror, hands on the wheel, and so on. Myra's voice calmed my monkey mind and convinced me I could actually do this. When she was confident that I was ready, she talked me through pulling away from the curb. We were off.

And I realize this is anticlimactic, but I felt…fine. Where we drove, there were very few cars. Myra watched me closely and approved. "You're a decent driver!" she exclaimed. "You're just a nervous and unpracticed driver." I felt absurdly pleased, the way I had when my father-in-law, a veterinarian, told me I had a very well-socialized cat. As we meandered through the shady streets, I felt no fear whatsoever. It was almost boring.

Cruise control

Of course, that first go-round, we'd kept things simple. At our second session, Myra and I drove on slightly busier streets. The time after that, we added the main drag, turns in traffic, and speed changes in and out of school zones. Each time I returned to Myra, my anxiety ramped up during the 24 hours leading up to the lesson. Then when I actually got behind the wheel, it mellowed out.

This fits with research showing that inexperienced skydivers' heart rates ratchet higher and higher until right after the moment they leap out the door of the plane, at which point their heart rates drop radically. In other words, the anticipation is by far the worst part. So says science! And Myra.

In practice, I found that I had the most anxiety when someone was tailing me closely, obviously annoyed with my rigorous respect for the speed limit. I'd be very concerned about the feelings and emotions of this anonymous irked person, but Myra wouldn't have it. "Stop worrying about him!" she would say. "Let him worry about him! You're following the law, and if he wants to pass you, he can pass you!"

Myra was smart about my anxiety. "The hardest moment for you," she observed, "is when you touch the outside door handle." She was right: I'd built up the notion of driving into this massive thing, and it had taken on a life of its own, one that had nothing to do with actually piloting a vehicle. In all the crashes I'd been in, I was a passenger—powerless. The fear of driving itself was what I'd been fearing, to lousily paraphrase FDR.

Guru Myra

I laughed when it dawned on me that almost everything Myra said in that car felt like a Zen koan that applied not only to driving but also to life: "Don't join the pack!" "Focus on the big picture!" "Leave yourself an out!" When she told me, "People drive their cars the way they live their lives," it helped me focus on how I pilot. Am I tentative and jumpy (or perhaps, worse, aggressive and bullying)? I want to be a generous driver and a generous person, someone who respects taking turns and takes reasonable risks.

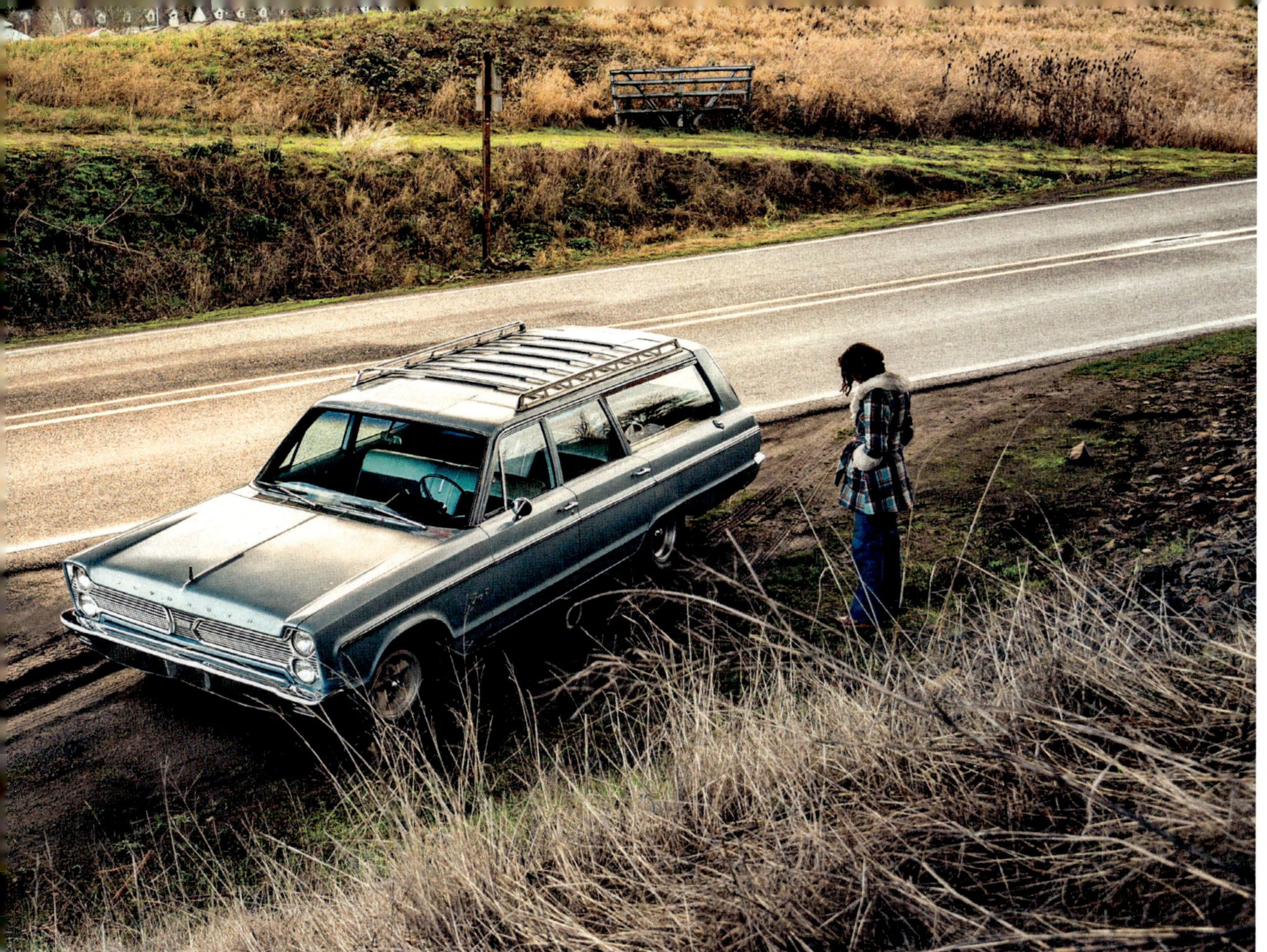

My takeaway from the advice "Be aware of blind spots" wasn't just to make sure a big truck could see me; it was to be aware of my own biases and blocks. My blind spot, as Myra had helped me realize, was that I was more paralyzed by the prospect of driving than by the act of driving. My husband had his own blind spot—that his tangible annoyance at me in the car made my anxiety in the car worse. We both had to tune in, focus, and work on vehicular growth and coexistence.

Then there was a classic: "Expect the unexpected," said Myra. Meaning, some schmuck could plow through a stop sign or a kid could chase a ball into the road, so don't get complacent. This sounds negative, but it needn't be. With a little practice, nervousness can be transmogrified into alertness. When you're attuned to your environment and open to possibility, you can be ready for adventure and more attentive to life's quirky moments—with your kids, your spouse, nature, a movie, a play, a physical sensation.

Road to somewhere

Ordinarily I am the person whose eyes roll like dice in a craps game when people say anything too woo-woo spiritual. Mystical clichés make me hork. But facing something that scared the living daylights out of me made me see these gems as truly meaningful. Yes, Myra's advice was meant to specifically improve my driving skills, but when applied to something that had legitimately been holding me back for years, it felt expansive and potent. And it made me view the future as full of possibility, independence, and action.

Driving really is about trusting yourself and being respectful of others without letting them dictate your behavior; you need the belief that you know what you're doing, which it's taking me a while to build. I still get a tiny stab of fear when I touch the car-door handle. And I haven't driven on the highway yet, though I feel confident that I can. But now I can picture myself driving—taking my kids to the Korean spa, going to that cult ice cream place in Tiverton, Rhode Island, visiting friends upstate.

Even if I never manage to, say, cruise down to Mexico in a convertible, hair blowing in the wind, one thing is for sure: I'm finally, after all these years, beginning to take the wheel. ●

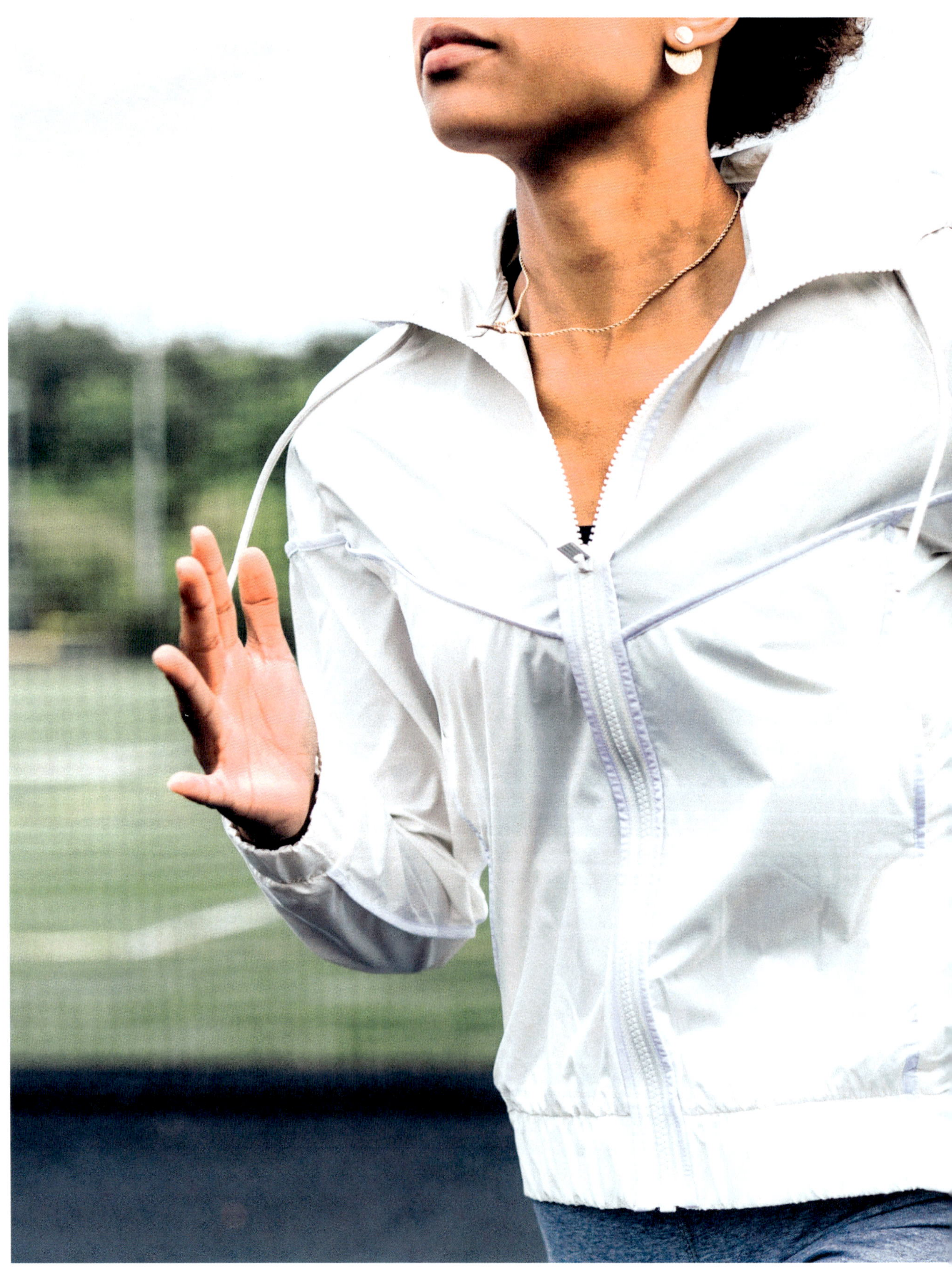

Mind and Body

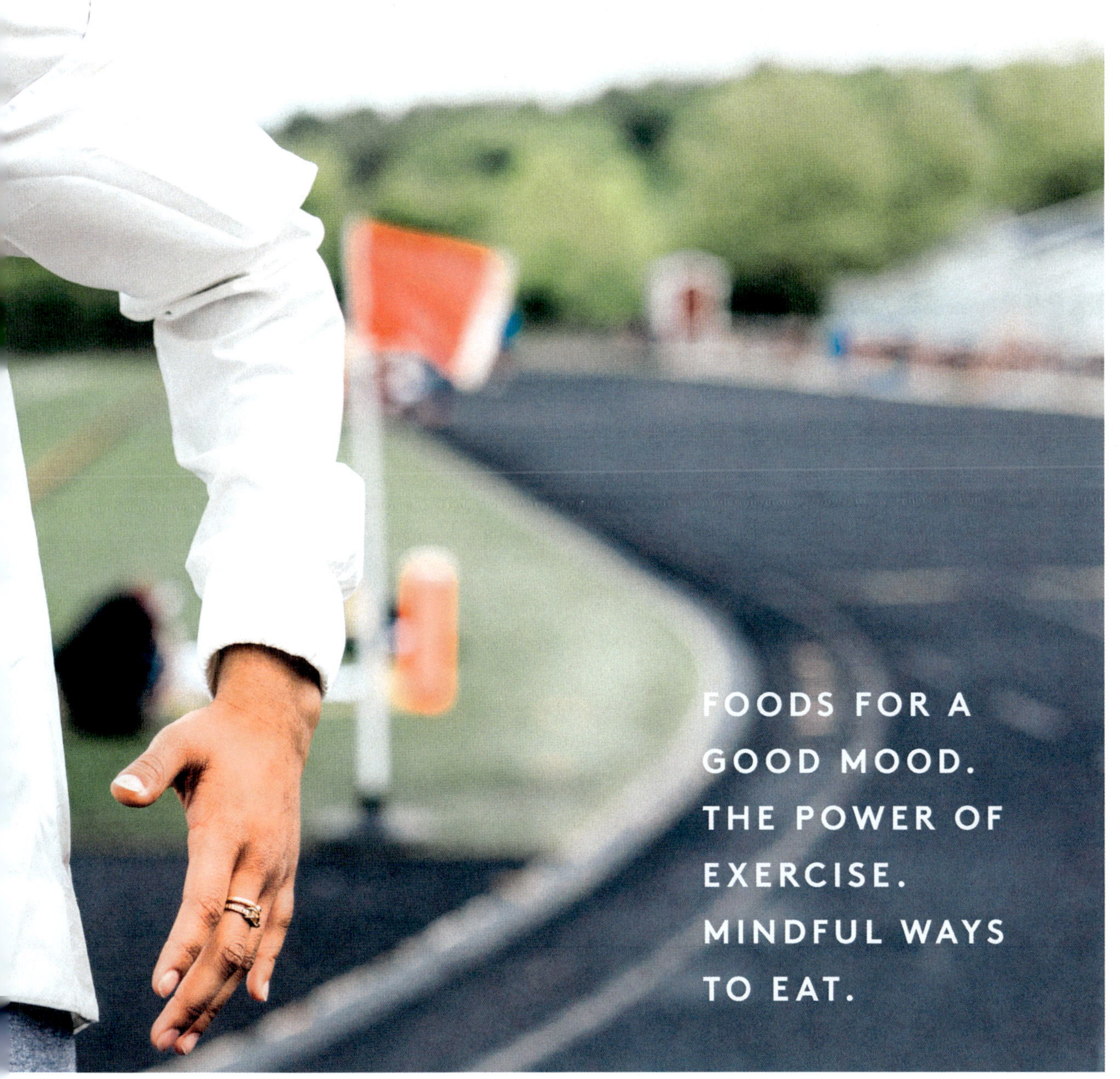

FOODS FOR A GOOD MOOD. THE POWER OF EXERCISE. MINDFUL WAYS TO EAT.

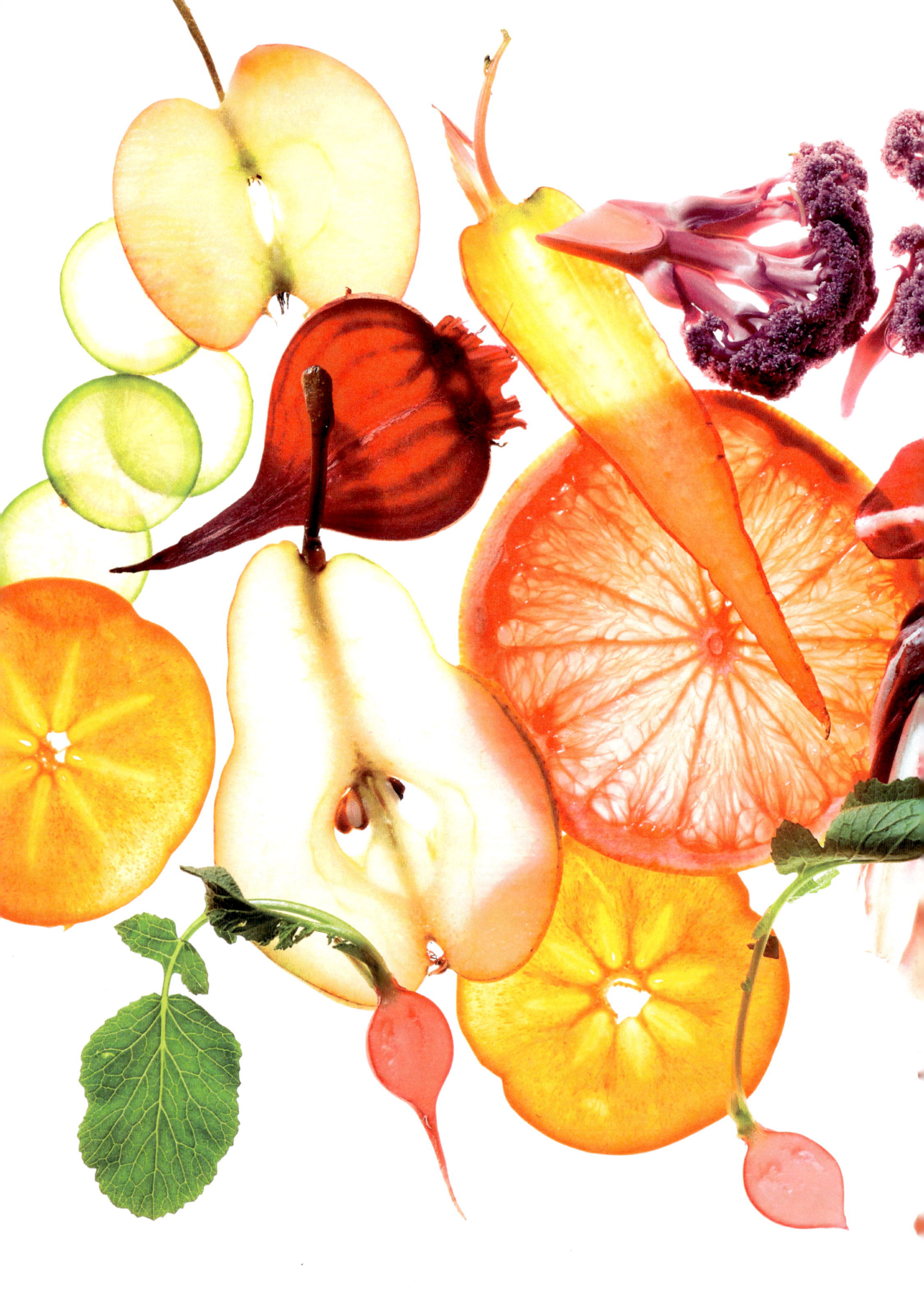

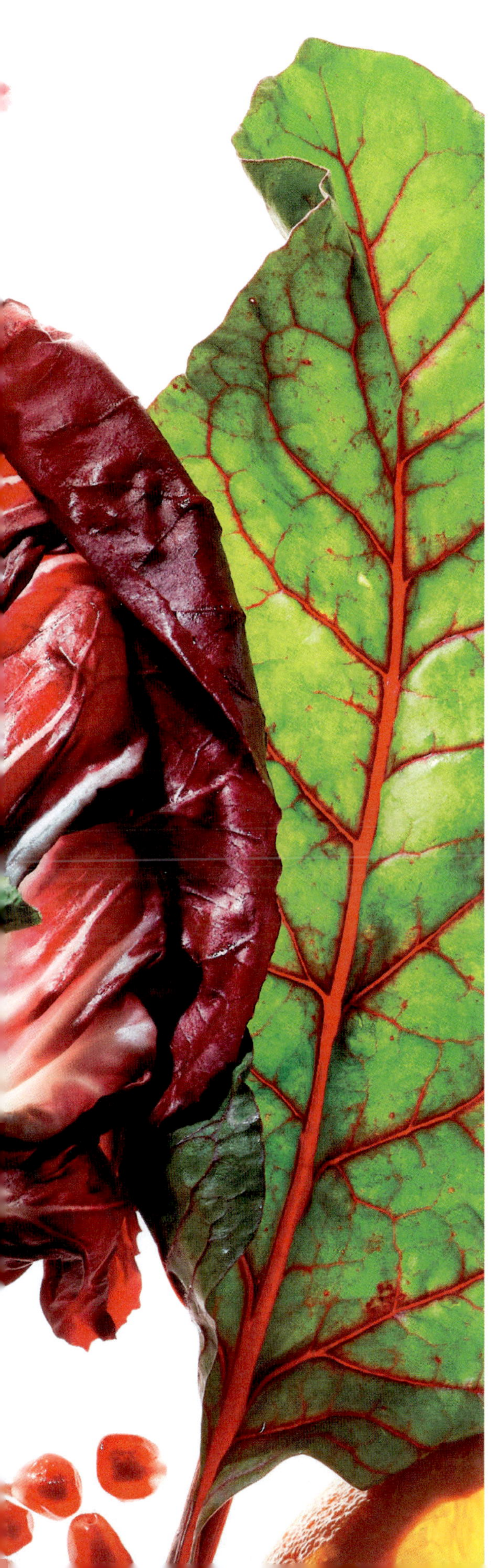

Feed Your (Great) Mood

EVERY DAY, EVERY MEAL, IS A NEW CHANCE TO FUEL YOUR BODY AND MIND.

By Sara Gaynes Levy

JUST WHEN YOU THOUGHT you'd mastered the essential art of self-care, here comes perhaps the easiest way to help create harmony in your day and improve your mood. Nope, it's not a mani-pedi or 20 minutes with a good book. Instead, you can eat your way to a happier you. Really.

What we eat each day affects us in countless ways, from fortifying our immune systems to aiding in heart health. But fueling your body with vitamins, minerals, and nutrients also helps boost your mood all day long. The approach, which combines the latest nutrition research and the expertise of dietitians, puts the power to get in a great headspace—and stay there—right on your plate. First and most important, you need to balance your protein, fat, and carbs in each meal and snack. Then schedule your sugar intake to help maintain mental focus. Finally, work in some gut-healthy foods to help keep anxiety at bay. Enhance your mood with the following feel-good guidelines.

To feel happy: Balance your macronutrients

You may have heard your CrossFit friends going on about "macros." These are the three main nutrients in food: protein, fat, and carbohydrates. Getting the right combination of macros at every meal does more than help prevent weight gain or make you feel full. "Stable blood sugar really helps put you in a good mood—and to get that, you want a balance of macronutrients," explains Sarah Dimitratos, RD, a PhD candidate in nutritional biology at the University of California, Davis. Don't worry: You can achieve this without counting calories or obsessively tracking what you eat. Just aim to fill half your plate with fruits and vegetables, a quarter with protein, and a quarter with whole-grain carbs. Work in some healthy fats by, say, roasting veggies in coconut oil or adding sliced avocado and—boom!—you've just balanced your macros. Also, try to get omega-3 fatty acids from foods like salmon, flaxseed, and hemp hearts. Omega-3s help maintain the nerves in the brain that are responsible for quick decision-making.

Keep balancing those macros throughout the day, each time you eat—ideally, every three to four hours. "If you want energy all day long, then you have to give your body energy all day long," says Tara Collingwood, a registered dietitian nutritionist in Orlando, Florida. Had breakfast at 6 a.m.? Plan on a snack around 10. Eating frequently can elevate your mood and help you avoid the unhappy feelings you experience when you're stuffed. "If you eat to get full, you might end up feeling groggy," Collingwood says. "If you eat small amounts more often, you feel sustained and energized." Research backs this up: Women who ate breakfast instead of skipping it were happier and more relaxed in the morning, one study found.

If your macros get out of whack—for example, because you only eat protein and/or fat—you might become cranky. "Carbs are your body's preferred source of energy. Mood and energy can be negatively affected when you're not eating carbs," says Collingwood, who suggests getting carbs from fruits, vegetables, and whole grains (as opposed to white-flour breads, muffins, and pretzels). However, if your meal or snack is too heavy in carbs—especially those refined white-flour carbs—your blood sugar can spike, then crash. You know what that's like: "It translates to lethargy, brain fog, irritability, and difficulty getting work done," Dimitratos says. In other words, you're not going to be happy.

To stay focused: Time your sugar right

It's a trap we often fall into. We enjoy a rich, sugary treat as an afternoon pick-me-up, which gives a quick boost and feels good while we're eating it. But it's worth keeping in mind what happens after you finish. "There's some evidence suggesting that the foods we tend to seek out under stress, which are really high in sugar, can create an inflammatory response in the body and brain," Dimitratos says. What's worse, as you give in to your sugar cravings, that midafternoon sweet becomes a habit—and it's hard to focus on work when all you're thinking about is snacking. (More bad news: Diets high in sugar and fat have been linked to more depression symptoms.)

You don't have to swear off sugar. Just understand its effects on you, and tune in to whether you're eating so much of it that you don't feel the way you'd like to. Collingwood's advice: "Pick moments when it doesn't matter what your energy level is." If it's been a long week and you just want to veg out, she says, that's the best time to have a sweet treat. "If you don't mind crashing on the couch with Netflix, then crash away!" On the other hand, she says, "if you have something important coming up, that's when you want to pay more attention to sugar and how much you're taking in." Got a big work presentation this afternoon? It's probably best to pass on the sweet stuff beforehand.

To keep calm: Try probiotics

Who among us hasn't felt that unpleasant stomach rumble during an anxious moment? The latest research indicates that the gut microbiome—the billions of good bacteria living in your digestive tract that influence everything from your body's ability to absorb nutrients to your immune system—has a direct line of communication to the brain. As such, our anxiety and stress can either lead to or result from gastrointestinal discomfort, creating a vicious

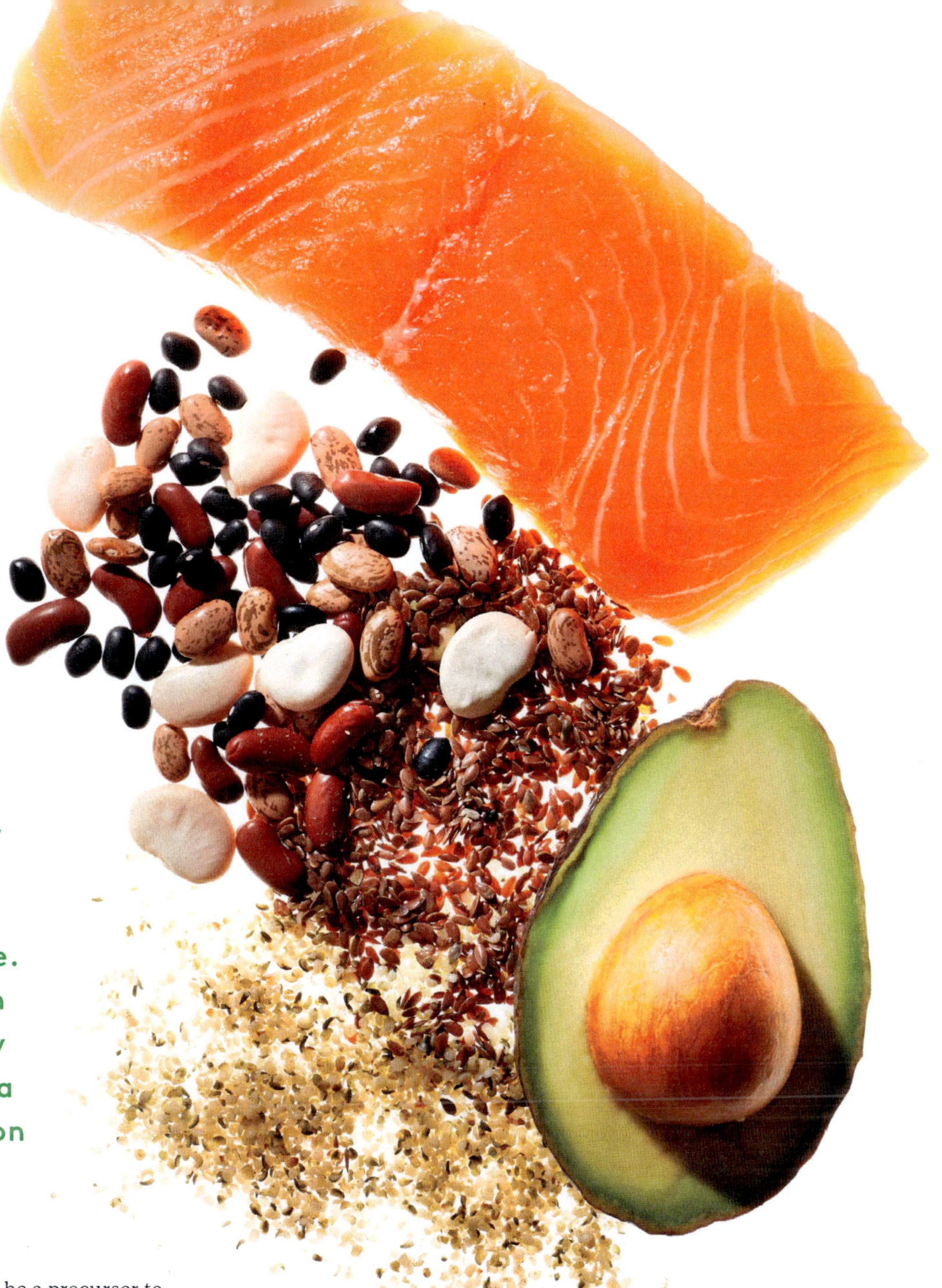

Probiotics may help reduce stress, anxiety, low moods, and mental fatigue. Think of them as the dietary equivalent of a daily meditation practice.

cycle. "Chronic stress can be a precursor to anxiety issues, and it's possible that chronic stress causes our intestinal lining to wear down," says Caroline Wallace, a PhD candidate at the Centre for Neuroscience Studies at Queen's University in Ontario, Canada, who studies probiotics and mental health. "Emerging research shows you can potentially use probiotics to help alleviate symptoms of anxiety and depression caused by chronic stress."

There's evidence that increasing your intake of probiotics can help ease negative GI symptoms. In turn, probiotics may help reduce stress, anxiety, low moods, and mental fatigue—common symptoms of depression. Think of them as the dietary equivalent of a daily meditation practice.

You can take probiotics in supplement form or eat probiotic-rich foods, like yogurt, sauerkraut, kimchi, and miso. It's still early, but "with regard to mental health, the studies are basically neutral or positive," Wallace says. "If you experience symptoms of depression or anxiety, be sure to see a professional, but there's no harm in also trying probiotics."

You have everything to gain and nothing to lose. ●

Habits That Are Secretly Making Us Irritable

MODERN LIFE—WITH ITS MISSED LUNCHES AND ROSÉ NIGHTCAPS—MESSES WITH OUR BRAINS AND MOODS IN POWERFUL WAYS. DON'T WORRY, IT'S ALL FIXABLE.

By Hallie Levine

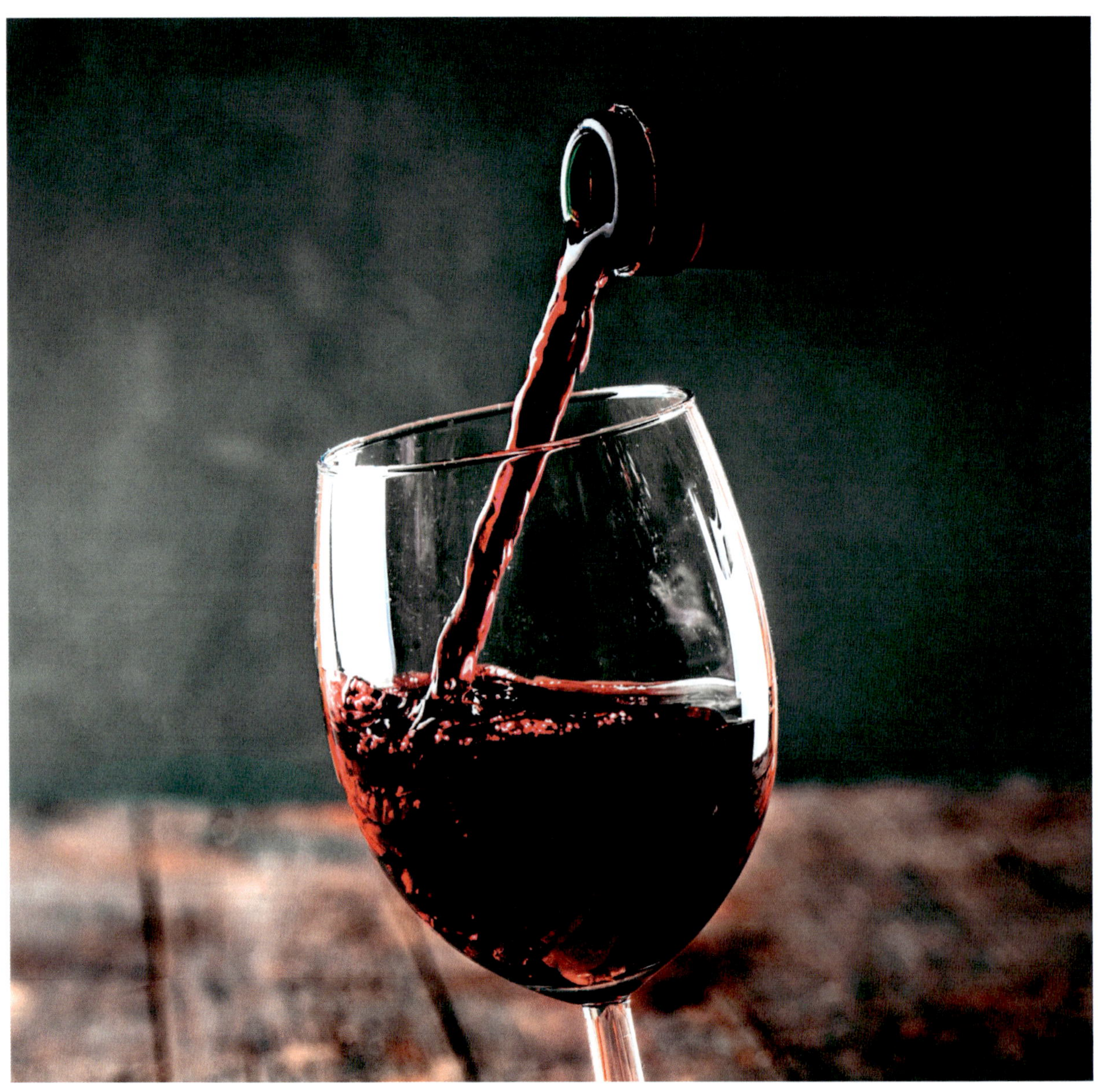

"Many people believe [alcohol] will help them sleep, but it disturbs your natural sleep patterns, so you're less likely to get that deep, quality sleep you need."

WALKING AROUND with a short fuse? You're not the only one. "We all face a certain amount of uncertainty and stress in our everyday lives, and sometimes that can manifest as irritability," says Mark Moyad, MD, MPH, the Jenkins/Pokempner director of preventive and alternative medicine at the University of Michigan. But the truth is that the smaller choices we make every day—how often we're on social media, what we eat and when, our alcohol and exercise habits, and even what we do during our downtime—can affect our moods more than we realize. Here, six habits that may secretly be making you cranky—and how to tweak them into ones that are better for your mental health.

You're snacking on the wrong foods

Whether you're stuck at your desk or at home, it's tempting to munch on chips or sugary granola bars. These aren't just bad for your waistline; they're bad for your mood too. A study published in 2020 in the *European Journal of Nutrition* looked at almost 15,000 people and found that those who ate the highest amounts of ultra-processed foods had a 33 percent higher risk of developing depression than those who included them minimally in their diet. "These foods tend to be lower in essential nutrients such as omega-3 fatty acids and B vitamins that play a crucial role in brain health," explains Samantha Heller, MS, RD, a nutritionist at New York University. Ultra-processed foods also tend to be low in fiber, which may affect your gut microbiome—the mix of good and bad bacteria in your gastrointestinal tract—which in turn negatively impacts your mood. The good bacteria in your gut produce a lot of neurotransmitters implicated in mood, like norepinephrine and GABA, notes Drew Ramsey, MD, a psychiatrist at Columbia University Medical Center and the author of *Eat to Beat Depression*. And while the mood-boosting hormone serotonin is usually thought of as a brain chemical, more than 90 percent of it is made in your GI tract, which is even more reason a healthy microbiome is important.

Your best bet is to fuel up on probiotic-rich snacks, such as Greek yogurt, kefir, or even cottage cheese, Ramsey advises. Include other probiotic picks, such as tofu, miso, kimchi, sauerkraut, and pickles, into your diet every day. And if you have a carb craving, reach for sourdough bread—it's baked with fermented flour that contains good bacteria.

You're drinking too close to bedtime

It's hard to wind down and relax after a long, stressful day, so it shouldn't come as a surprise that many of us are turning to a nightcap—or two or three—to help us nod off. In March 2020, alcoholic-beverage sales in stores were up 54 percent (over the previous year), and online sales soared well over 400 percent throughout April, according to data from the Nielsen Corporation. "Many people believe it will help them sleep, but it disrupts your natural sleep patterns, so you're less likely to get that deep, quality sleep you need," explains Dean Drosnes, MD, the medical director of the Pennsylvania Caron Treatment Center. Even moderate consumption of alcohol can impair your restorative sleep quality by 24 percent, according to a 2018 study in the *Journal of Mental Health*. This in turn can make you irritable. "Alcohol is a [central-nervous-system] depressant anyway, so it can worsen symptoms of depression and anxiety," adds Drosnes. You don't need to give up your daily cocktail, but Drosnes suggests having it earlier in the evening—around dinner time—and limiting yourself to just one.

You're spending too much time on social media feeds

Research increasingly shows that the more time you spend scrolling on sites like Facebook and Instagram, the greater your risk of depression. In fact, a 2018 University of Pennsylvania study published in the *Journal of Social and Clinical Psychology* found that college students who limited their time on Facebook, Instagram and Snapchat to just 10 minutes a day reported significant decreases in depression and loneliness compared with those who didn't. "These sites can foster all sorts of unhealthy comparisons to others, especially if they're posting photos of their so-called fabulous life and you already feel crummy," says Bruce Rabin, MD, PhD, a professor emeritus of pathology at the University of Pittsburgh and the director of the Healthy Lifestyle Program at the University of Pittsburgh Medical Center.

They can also invite a news cycle into your life 24/7, which in turn can leave you depressed and anxious. "I recommend my patients schedule a time to check emails, scroll through social media, or watch the news," says Leela Magavi, MD, a regional medical director for Community Psychiatry in Newport Beach, California. Otherwise, you'll find yourself scrolling at all hours of the day, including in the wee hours of the night, which can impact sleep length and quality and definitely worsen irritability. And try to take some of that extra time you used to spend on social media on another activity, such as volunteering. People who volunteer regularly have better health outcomes, including lower rates of anxiety and depression, than those who don't, according to a 2017 review published in *BMC Public Health*.

You're skimping on physical activity

Ever wonder why you're especially grumpy when you haven't had a sweat session in a few days? Blame it on being sedentary. "It lowers levels of feel-good brain hormones such as serotonin, which can cause you to feel angry and irritable," says Moyad. You don't need to do much to feel better: A single bout of exercise is enough to increase levels of feel-better brain hormones such as endogenous opioids and endocannabinoids (these are responsible for the so-called runner's high). If you're having trouble squeezing in regular workouts, Moyad recommends focusing on slipping in little bursts of activity throughout the day. "All those basic household chores like sweeping, vacuum cleaning, gardening, dusting, washing windows, ironing, making beds, laundry, washing dishes, and stair climbing can potentially address fitness deficits," he says.

You're skipping lunch

Almost three-quarters of Americans no longer eat three square meals a day, according to a 2018 survey by market research provider OnePoll. The main meal that's fallen by the wayside now is lunch, with almost half saying they substitute it with some small snacks instead. But opting out of a midday meal is a recipe for disaster, says Cordialis Msora-Kasago, MA, RDN, a spokesperson for the Academy of Nutrition and Dietetics in Menifee, California. "It causes your blood sugar to plummet, and since there's not enough glucose for your brain to function well, you end up feeling irritable, confused, and fatigued," she explains. In addition, your body may ramp up its production of the stress hormone cortisol as an emergency response, leaving you feeling even more stressed and grouchy. Ideally, you want to space meals and snacks out evenly through the day so you're eating every three to four hours, says Msora-Kasago. This will help keep blood sugar levels stable and prevent that "hangry" feeling.

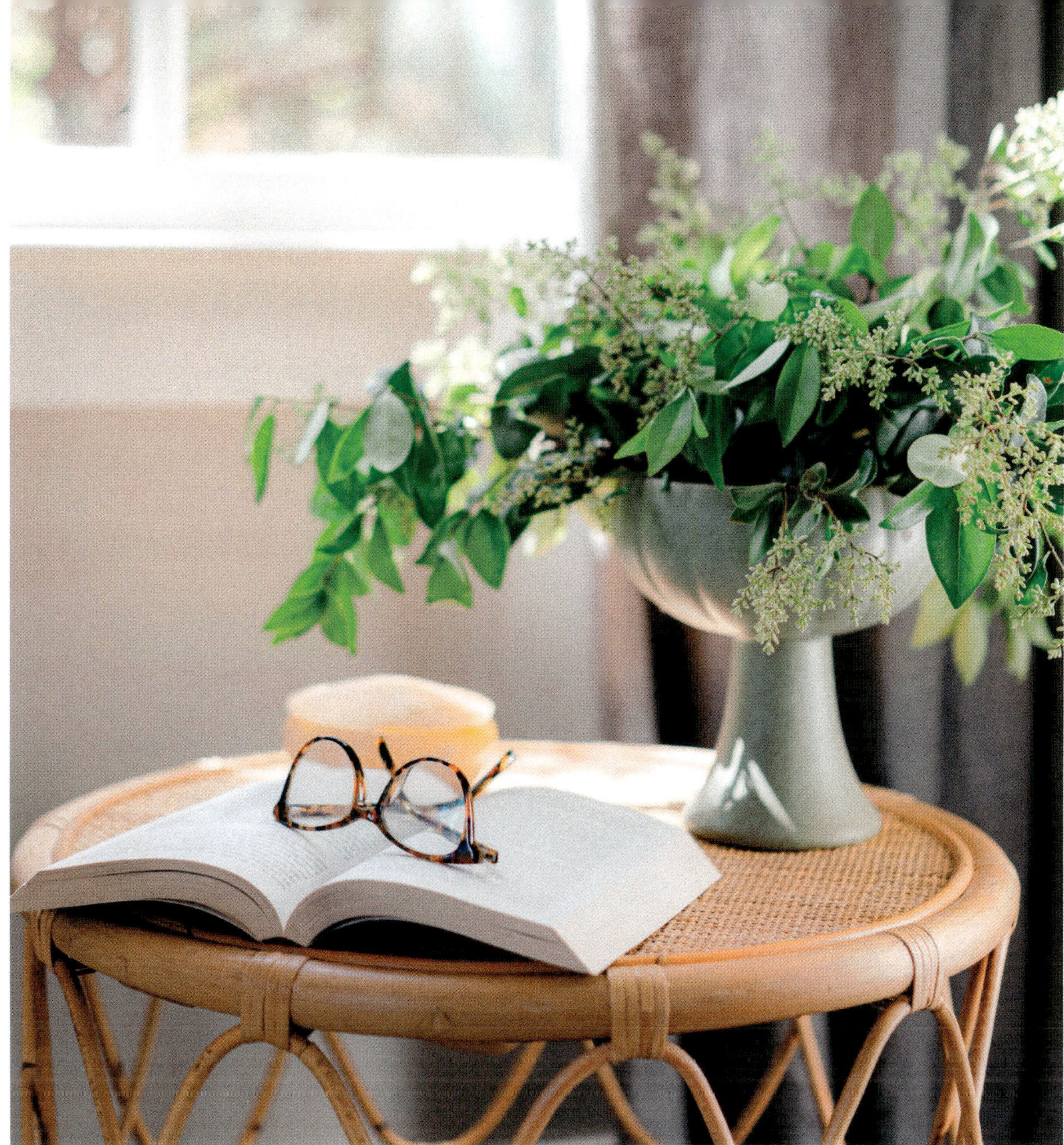

You forget to give yourself some love

In a May 2020 survey from the nonprofit organization LeanIn.org, a quarter of women reported experiencing physical symptoms of severe anxiety such as a racing heartbeat. Half complained of sleep issues, and almost a third said they were just more overwhelmed in general. But this is a path that leads to burnout and general resentment. "It takes a lot of initiative and planning to make time for ourselves, but if we don't carve it out, it doesn't come," says Erin Murray, MS, a nutritionist and health coach in Boston. Aim to do something that's just for you every day, whether it's taking time to pick up ingredients so you can cook yourself something you love, setting aside a few extra minutes to read a great book, or taking the evening completely off to binge-watch *Ozark*. "When we have no time to reflect and recover mentally, our ego gets grumpy," Murray adds. Another mood-changing option: doing three minutes of meditation, such as deep-breathing exercises. A 2014 review of 47 studies published in *JAMA Internal Medicine* found that mindfulness-meditation programs improved symptoms of anxiety and depression. ●

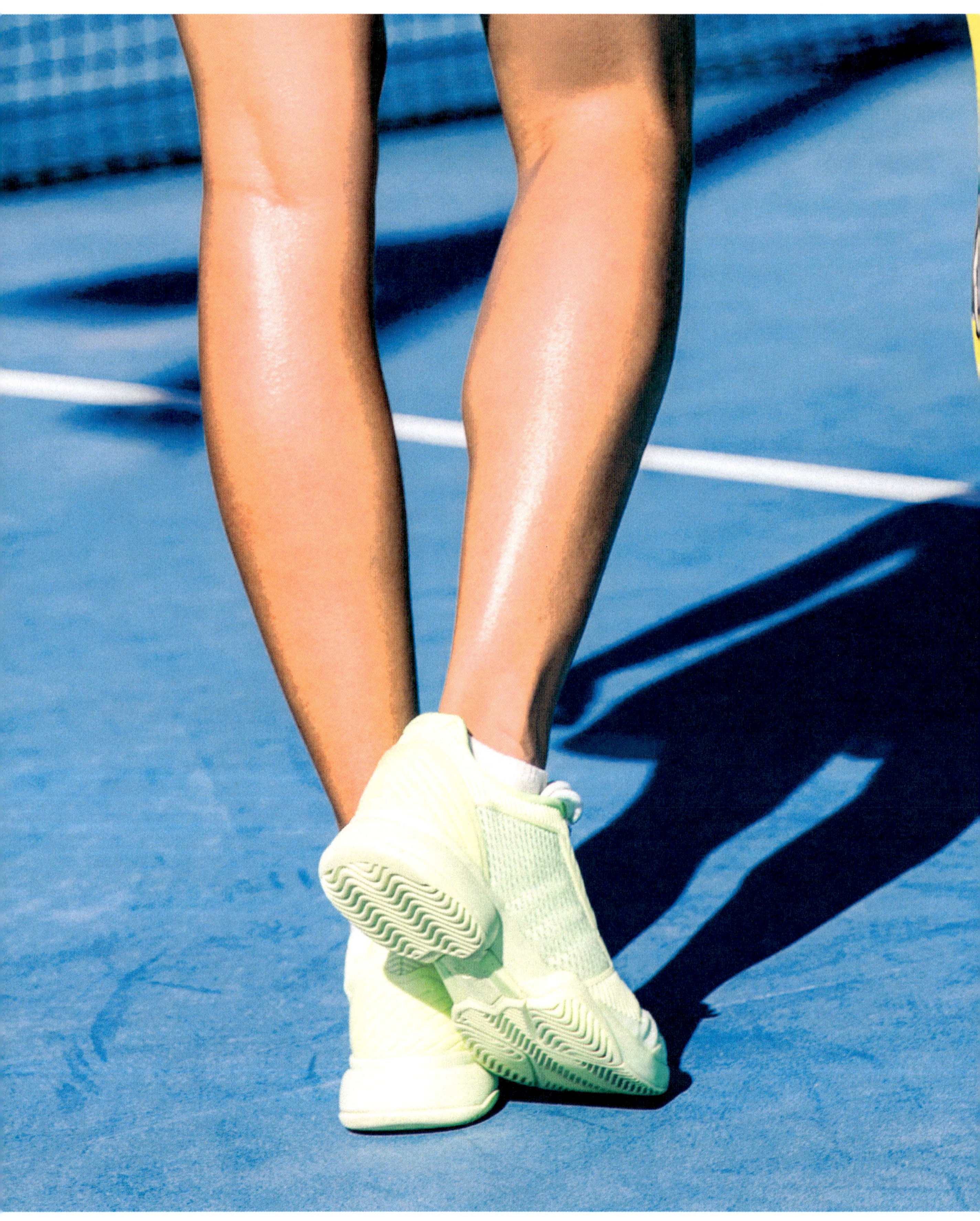

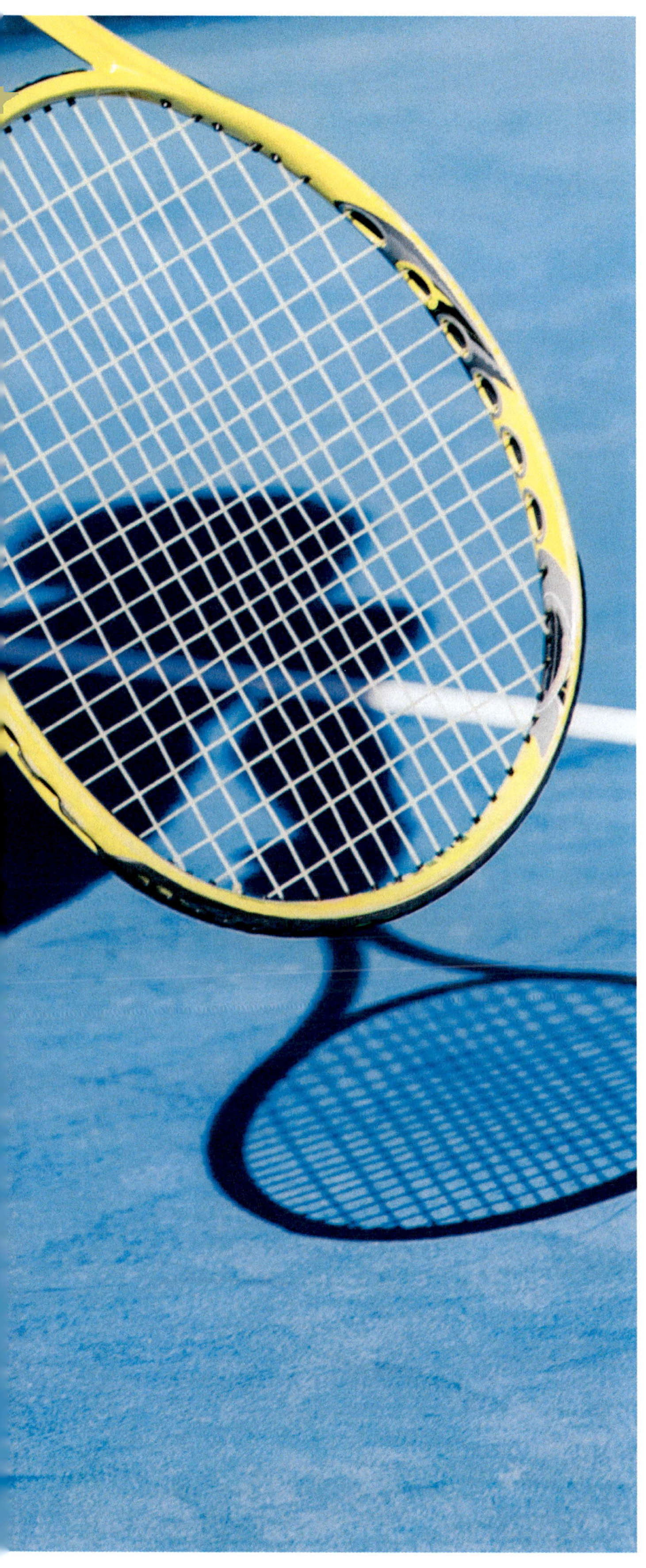

Work Out, Feel the Joy

REASON NO. 781 TO EXERCISE: IT BATHES YOUR BRAIN IN MOOD-BOOSTING CHEMICALS.

By Leslie Goldman

IN 2002, WENDY SUZUKI, PHD, was a New York University neuroscientist with a focus on human memory. Long hours spent sitting in a lab weren't doing her fitness level or social life any favors, so she signed up for a river-rafting trip in Peru. Once there, she discovered she was the weakest person in the group, and she returned home determined to get in shape, joining a gym and hiring a personal trainer.

After fumbling through her first hip-hop dance session ("I was so bad!" she says), Suzuki noticed something: "I felt energized and satisfied that I had made it through that difficult class." Motivated by the mood and energy lift, she kept at it. More benefits racked up: enhanced memory, sharper focus. A year and a half later, she shifted the focus of her research to exercise's ability to strengthen and rewire the brain. Suzuki published research highlighting the ability of a single workout to elevate mood for up to 24 hours and even started teaching aerobics classes. Her TED Talk, "The Brain Changing Benefits of Exercise," has been viewed nearly 10 million times.

We've all heard about (or, depending on our activity level, personally enjoyed) the coveted runner's high. But you don't need to wear holes in your gym shoes to experience the stress-busting, mood-bumping effects of exercise. Suzuki, now a professor of neural science and psychology at New York University, says the benefits of regular workouts are available to anyone regardless of fitness level or access to a gym; can be as effective as antidepressants in some people; and, over the long term, act like "401(k) deposits to maximize mood."

Here's how a little heart-pumping action can be your smartest investment in your mental health.

Exercise delivers a lasting mood boost

Whether you're briskly walking through your neighborhood, riding a stationary bike, playing tennis, or taking a yoga class, you're unwittingly kicking off a neurochemical cascade that steeps your brain in feel-great neurotransmitters like dopamine, noradrenaline, and serotonin (the same chemical messenger targeted by many antidepressants). The cascade is thought to be triggered by your rising heart rate, and the effects are powerful and swift. Cedric X. Bryant, PhD, the president and chief science officer of the American Council on Exercise, says you can expect to feel a hit of happy after just five minutes of moderate-intensity exercise. (Moderate-intensity means your heart is pumping and you may be a bit out of breath but can still comfortably have a conversation.)

As dopamine increases, so do growth factors that stimulate the birth of new cells in the hippocampus, a seahorse-shaped region of the brain charged with forming new memories as well regulating mood. Imagine bathing your brain in those spirit-sustaining chemicals week after week, month after month. "Now you're not just getting a little blip of improved mood after a workout," Suzuki says, "but you're changing your baseline mood from lower to higher." A 2019 *JAMA Psychiatry* study led by Karmel Choi, PhD, a clinical and research fellow at the Harvard T.H. Chan School of Public Health and Massachusetts General Hospital, found that the impact can be strong enough to lower the risk of depression. Researchers reviewed genetic data from more than 600,000 adults and discovered that those who completed the daily equivalent of 15 minutes of vigorous activity (like running) or an hour of moderately paced activity (like fast walking) were 26 percent less likely to develop depression.

When studying the link between exercise and mood, scientists often bring up the chicken-or-egg nature of the relationship: Does exercise truly protect against mood, or do happier people tend to be more active? Choi says that by employing high-level analytic techniques using genetic information, she and her colleagues found evidence of a causal relationship in only one direction, suggesting that exercise does reduce the odds of depression, not the other way around.

Another happy side effect of exercise is that it tuckers you out, and good, quality sleep boasts a rock-solid tie with improved mood. "We know that sleep deprivation, like that caused by stress, staying up late in front of screens, or drinking caffeine in the afternoon, causes irritability, anger, and depression," says Sara C. Mednick, PhD, the director of the Sleep and Cognition Lab at the University of California, Irvine. "But consistently getting around eight hours of sleep can help reverse those effects, bathing your brain in serotonin and leading to a more positive long-term outlook." People who engage in regular aerobic activity fall asleep faster, spend more time in deep sleep, and wake fewer times in the middle of the night.

Movement is an antidote to stress

Consistent exercise can also act as a soothing stress balm. This might be the result of pain-relieving endorphins produced during a workout, which foster a sense of well-being and an "I got this" attitude, or it could simply be that getting your sweat on distracts you from the stressors of daily life. "When you're running, you focus on your breathing or your stride frequency and length, and that helps provide that distraction," Bryant says. Recreational sports like tennis and golf "can be even more powerful because you get caught up in the game" instead of thinking about career pressure, financial woes, or whatever else may be causing you anxiety.

Moving your body through a

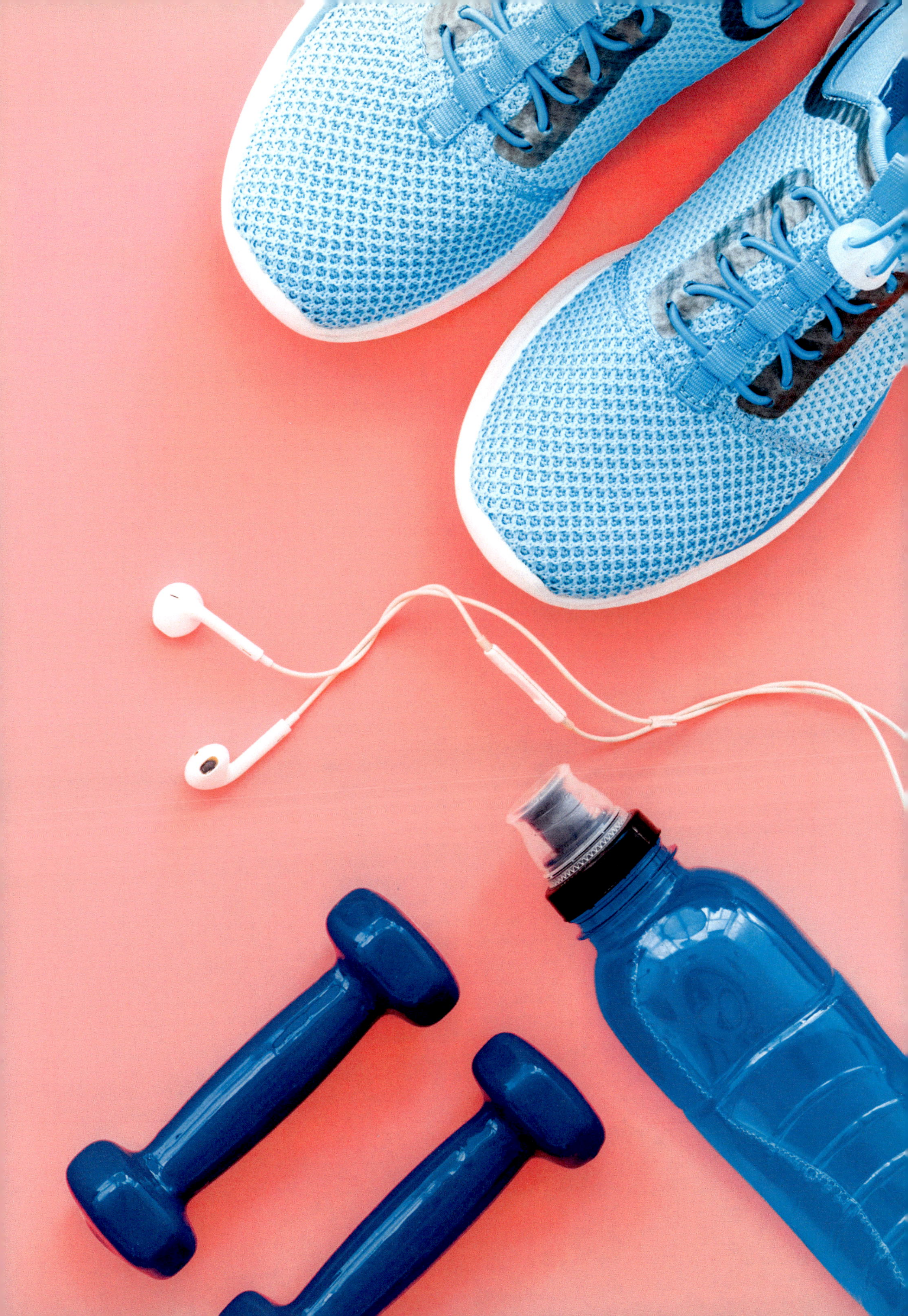

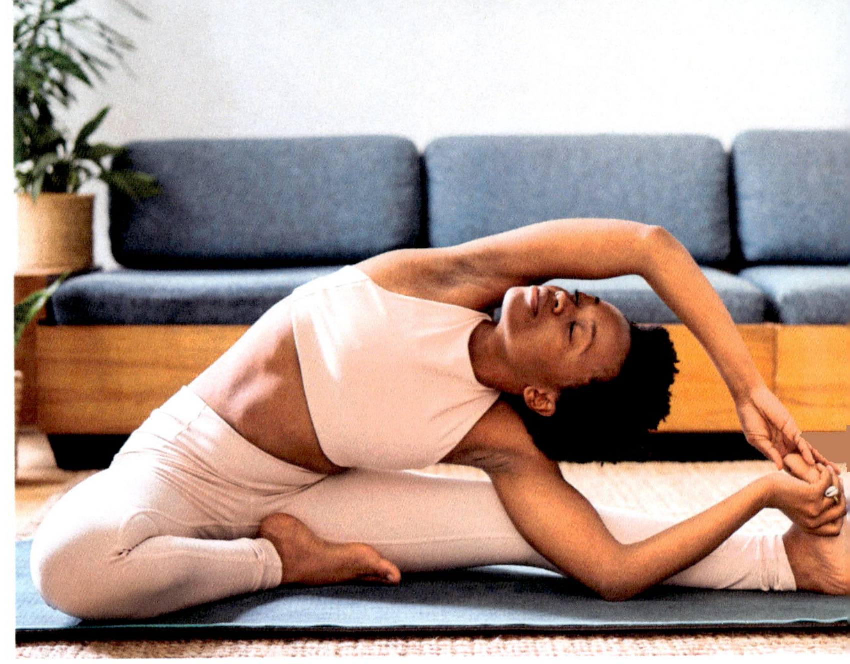

workout may also alleviate stress by teaching your brain that if you can get through this tricky yoga pose or final mile of jogging, you can get through other challenges in life. "Exercise may be a form of controlled, predictable stress that, when you willingly put yourself through it, you learn that you can handle tough challenges," says Choi, who is also a clinical psychologist.

Finally, cutting-edge research suggests that physical activity can invigorate our mental outlook by balancing the two branches of the nervous system, the sympathetic (fight-or-flight) and parasympathetic (rest-and-digest). In most of us, chronic stress causes the sympathetic nervous system to dominate. But during exercise, Mednick says, "you can have an extreme rise in heart rate as your body mobilizes its resources to get blood pumped out to your extremities." (That's the sympathetic system in action.) When the workout ends, your body works hard to bring your cardiovascular and muscular systems back to their normal resting state. In the process, it decreases levels of a stress hormone called cortisol and releases those lovely neuroprotective hormones. The result: better nervous system balance, less stress, upgraded mood.

The bottom line: As you build and sculpt your muscles, you're simultaneously building and sculpting the mood-regulating portion of your brain.

And the amount of exercise you need is...

Now for the question that Suzuki says everyone loves to ask: What is the minimum amount of exercise needed to reap all of these rewards?

Different studies have yielded different findings. Australian and German sports sociology experts found that recreational athletes who met the World Health Organization's exercise guidelines (150 minutes of moderate physical activity per week) tended to experience better mental health than those who didn't. Bryant echoes these guidelines, endorsing 30 minutes of moderate-intensity activity on most days of the week. But in a recent *American Journal of Psychiatry* study in which nearly 34,000 adults were followed for 11 years, researchers estimated that 12 percent of cases of depression could have been prevented if everyone had dedicated just one hour a week to physical activity of any intensity.

"If you are just starting your exercise journey, even a 15-minute power walk is enough to start to reap the benefits," Suzuki says. Remember, the goal is to get your heart rate up, so depending on your starting fitness level, that could be anything from a power walk to a boot-camp video.

And while it might seem counterintuitive, harder is not necessarily better. "Try to stay at the point where you can talk," Bryant says. Evidence exists that as you pass that threshold, you delay the immediate mood-boosting effect of the workout.

Choi's findings support the "less is more" philosophy in another way: Her study found that in addition to formal exercise, daily physical movement—think taking the stairs, putting away your laundry, or using a standing desk—"can add up to keep depression at bay. You might need to do more of it to get to the level that results in a 26 percent decrease in depression risk, but it still helps." •

A NEUROSCIENTIST'S FAVORITE WORKOUT

When neuroscientist Wendy Suzuki started her exercise journey, she took a class called intenSATI. It pairs high-intensity dance cardio with yoga, martial arts, and affirmations. ("I am strong now!" "Yes I can!") You don't need to become a certified intenSATI instructor like Suzuki did to feel all those feels. Just repeat a mantra as you run. *Yes, you can!*

I Found Surprising Peace Through Running

A reluctant athlete started jogging to get in shape—and found the calmness and clarity she craved.

By Holly Robinson

"You're not running today, are you?" My husband nodded toward the bruised rain clouds.

"Don't worry," I said. "I'll be fine." I laced up my sneakers and set off.

We were in England, staying near the Kennet and Avon Canal. The last time we'd been there, many years before, we'd explored the canal. Back then, watching a woman jog by, ponytail bouncing, I thought, "It must be nice to be able to run like that." Now here I was, running that same path. My ponytail days are over, but I wore a bright headband and tights. I almost couldn't believe it was me.

Ever since I'd started juggling motherhood and a job, I had little time for workouts. I wheezed like a bulldog when I climbed stairs. Shortly before my 60th birthday, I saw an ad for a Couch to 5K program. I assumed it was too expensive but emailed the coach anyway.

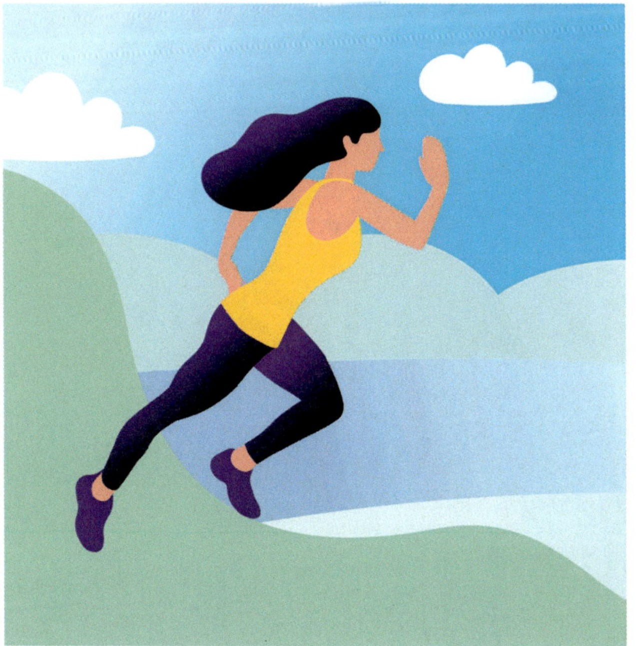

"It's free!" she wrote back.

"I'm 59. Isn't that too old?" I responded.

"I'm 70," she replied.

Good Lord. So I dug out a pair of sweats and drove to practice. To my relief, most of the other participants couldn't run a lap around the track either. Despite my legs and lungs begging me to quit, I stuck it out.

And after eight weeks, I ran a 5K. Two years later, I ran my first 10K. This was an achievement—but it wasn't as important as the discovery that running pauses the world around me. I began running trails instead of roads. Occasionally I startle wild turkeys and deer. Once I spotted an owl watching me from a branch. One route leads me into salt marshes, where egrets and herons feed.

Running has also been the best salve for emotional turmoil. It got me through my grief after my father-in-law died, and my sorrow after my youngest child left for college. In Virginia Woolf's *Moments of Being*, she describes nonbeing as "a kind of nondescript cotton wool." We're on autopilot. Being happens during those rare times when we're fully conscious of our surroundings and feel connected to them. We're all guilty of too many hours of nonbeing. Various tasks fracture our time, tech fills our heads with noise, and we stop paying attention to anything beyond ourselves. When I run, I have to pay attention. Running lets me be completely in the world, noticing small details, experiencing the joy of moving through snowflakes so big, it's like floating through lace.

Along the English towpath that recent morning, I flushed pheasants out of bushes and passed brightly painted boats. After five miles, it started to rain as I ran by a man in a tweed cap and rubber boots. He smiled and waved.

I waved back, and I thought about how we were sharing this moment. To him, I was a woman in a bright headband, admiring the dizzying patterns of early morning rain on the river. ●

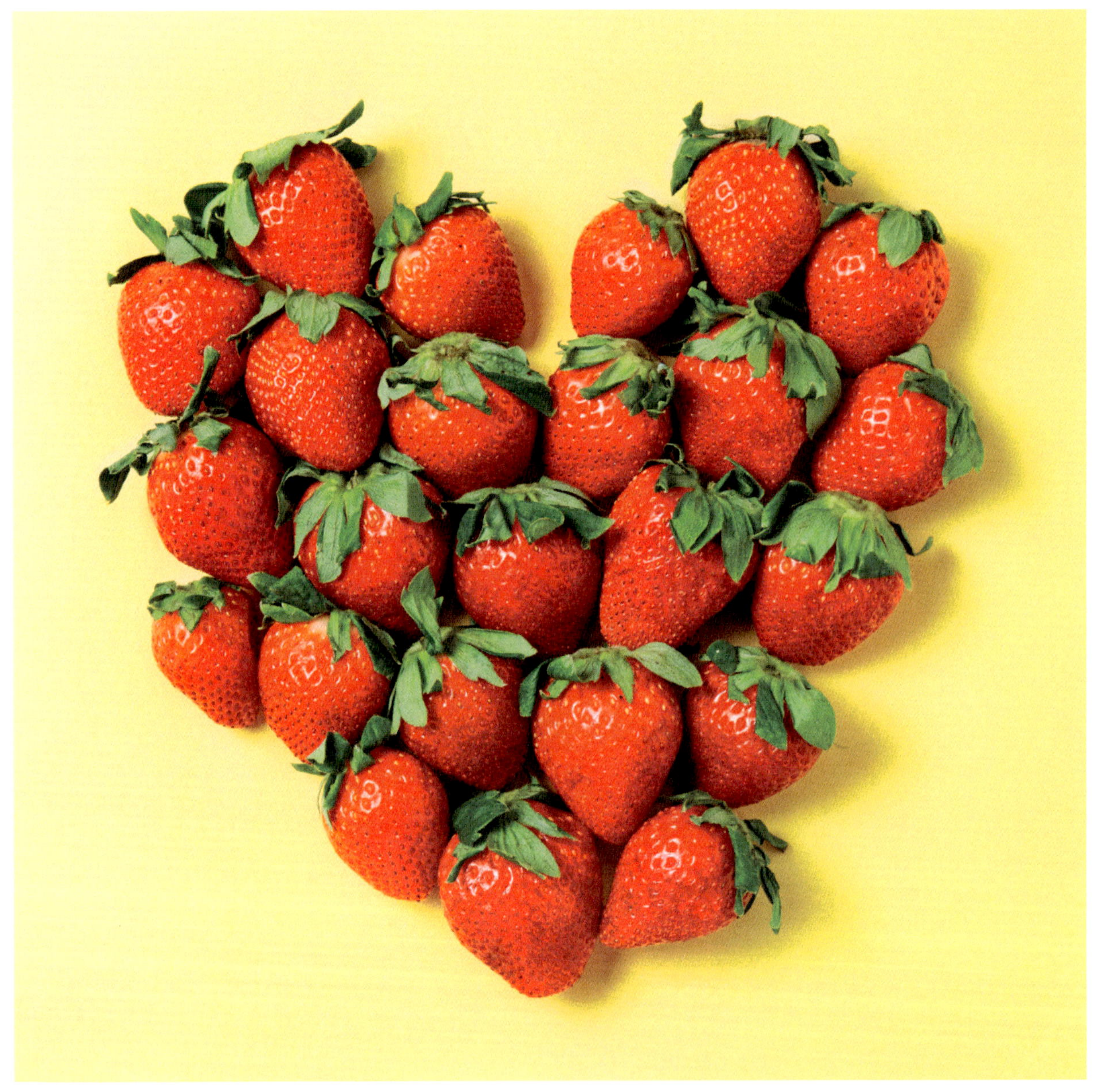

A Happier Way to Eat

INTUITIVE EATING—LISTENING TO OUR BODY'S HUNGER CUES—CAN REPAIR OUR GUILT-RIDDEN RELATIONSHIPS WITH FOOD AND OUR BODIES.

By Sharon Holbrook

WHAT IF WE told you that you can eat whatever you want and still be healthy? That there are no "good" or "bad" foods? That you never have to feel guilty about enjoying ice cream on a hot summer day or a slice of pie at a family gathering? You might think we were reporting on a new fad diet, but happily, the opposite is true. It was 25 years ago that two nutritionists unveiled a radical approach to food and health called intuitive eating—and it's now finally being embraced by the mainstream.

"People are tired of feeling at war with their own bodies," says Evelyn Tribole, RDN, who, with Elyse Resch, RDN, coauthored *Intuitive Eating*, a 10-principle approach that includes back-to-seriously-basic stuff: Pay attention to signals of hunger and fullness, reject diet mentality and food rules, and adopt body-positive behaviors, like exercising and eating food that makes you feel good.

The time is right for this approach to take hold. Only about 20 percent of women feel "very" or "extremely" satisfied with their weight, according to research in the journal *Body Image*. But even as the focus on dieting to be thin has given way to an emphasis on eating "clean" to be healthy, the obesity levels in our country have risen. Restricting food doesn't seem to be working. Exercising without changing our diets isn't effective either. Intuitive eating just might be the answer.

"There's been a backlash to all the rules about eating clean, which has created a space for intuitive eating," says Virginia Sole-Smith, the author of *The Eating Instinct: Food Culture, Body Image, and Guilt in America*. "It's less work, you give yourself permission to eat a range of foods, and you free yourself from weight-loss expectations."

How it works

Intuitive eating separates the idea of "healthy weight" from overall health. Research finds that people who engage in four habits—doing regular physical activity, eating at least five fruits and vegetables a day, not smoking, and consuming alcohol moderately—experience similar mortality rates, regardless of how much they weigh, says Kristen Murray, a registered dietitian in Cleveland, Ohio, who specializes in intuitive eating. Unlike dieting, which tends to be about restricting ourselves and trying to override our bodies' instincts, intuitive eating is about self-compassion and trusting our bodies, she says.

"I help people learn how to move away from the external cues telling them what, when, and how much to eat," she explains, "and get in touch with their internal cues telling them what, when, and how much to eat."

While it might sound too good to be true—permission to indulge in sugar whenever we feel like it?—there's evidence that intuitive eating works. As people reject restrictive food rules, they find that junk-food binges lose their rebellious appeal and that nutritious foods (proteins, whole grains, vegetables) are satisfying and make their bodies feel better. "More than 100 studies show that intuitive eating offers a multitude of health benefits," says Tribole. People who scored high on an Intuitive Eating Scale had higher body and life satisfaction and better coping skills. (People with low scores reported more eating-disorder symptoms and less satisfaction with their bodies.) Intuitive eating is also associated with increased optimism, psychological hardiness, and a greater motivation to exercise for pleasure, a recent review of 24 studies found. "We tend to think, 'Health is physical, and it's about your weight,'" says Rebecca Scritchfield, RDN, the author of *Body Kindness*. "But health is really about well-being."

This approach could not be more natural, but it might take time and patience to fully get the hang of it. Or get the hang of it again. Babies are born

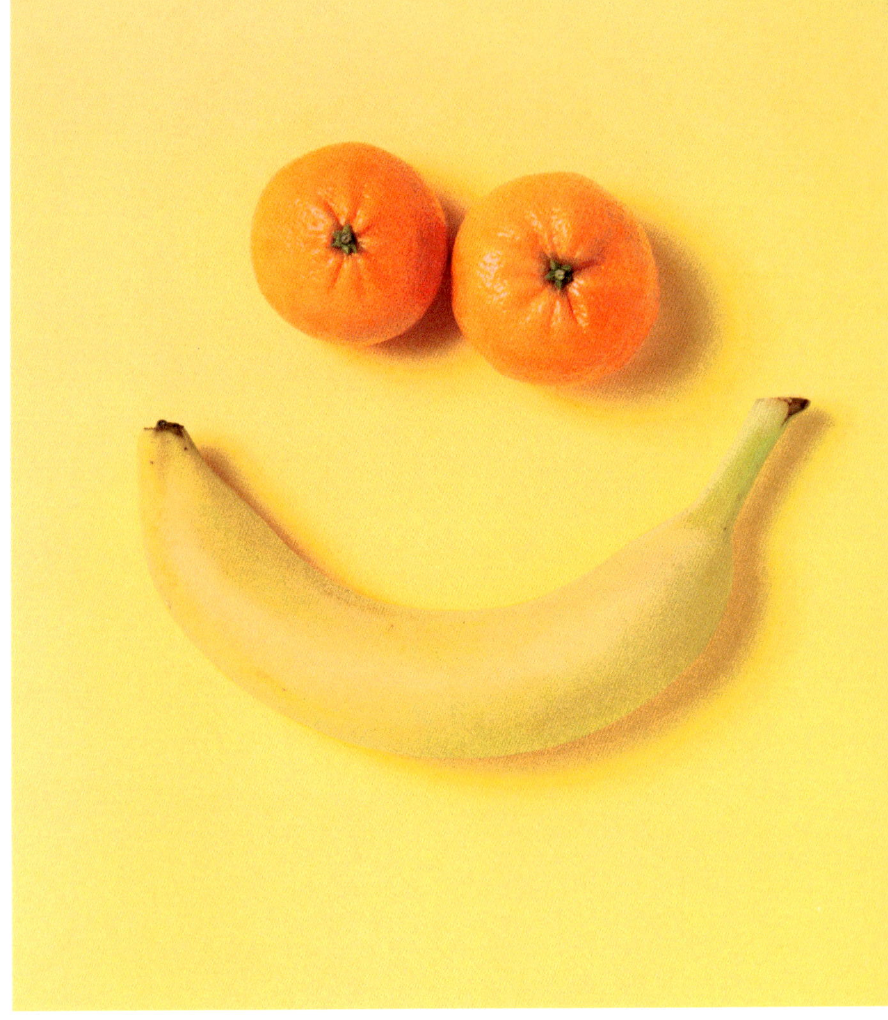

knowing to eat when they're hungry and stop when they're full—but our culture distorts these cues. "They get drowned out by diet messages and food marketing messages and guilt and relationships and access and so many other reasons," says Sole-Smith. "I don't think it's easy, but I do believe it's possible to reconnect with your instincts."

The following pillars of intuitive eating offer a few expert-backed ways to begin.

Be kind to your body

It can be challenging to treat yourself well (and feel good about doing so) if you've long considered your weight to be the first and best measure of your health, says Scritchfield. "Well-being is a blend of physical and mental health, and we're better off when we don't use weight as a measure," she says. It's normal to doubt that you will ever let go of weight ideals and accept your body. But if you succeed, an afternoon walk becomes about taking a break to clear your head and reboot your energy, rather than about burning a certain number of calories.

TRY THIS: Scritchfield suggests focusing on three aspects of body kindness: love, connection, and care. *Love* means choosing to love yourself even if you wish your body were different. *Connection* means being on the same team as your body; like a friend, you pay attention to what your body needs. *Care* means making choices based on that love and connection. For example, you can think about exercise in the following way: "I love my body, and while I may feel out of shape, I appreciate that it carries me through each day." Or "I connect with my body when I hear it tell me that it's hard to get up from the floor and that exercise might make me stronger, more flexible, and energized." Or "I care for my body by trying a YouTube yoga flow. Not because I need to whip my body into shape, but because I want to give it what it needs to feel good." By starting with body kindness, says Scritchfield, you'll reach a point when you make healthy physical and emotional choices that align with your goals.

We tend to think, "Health is physical, and it's about your weight." But health is really about well-being.

Listen to your body's signals

The next step is noticing and responding to hunger and feelings of fullness—which are truly at the heart of intuitive eating. Many of us are used to suppressing our bodies' messages, and not just about food. We work through lunchtime because we need to get a task done or want to lose weight. We watch yet another show on Netflix, not acknowledging that our bodies and brains are exhausted and it's time to sleep. We don't take a walk after sitting for hours at our desks, because we haven't stopped to think about how stiff and sluggish we are from a sedentary day.

TRY THIS: Set an alarm for every few hours and check in with your body. Give yourself credit for easy wins, like noticing whether you are warm or cold or need to use the restroom. This is what Tribole and Resch call "cultivating attunement." When you eat, remove distractions (turn off the TV, put away your phone) so you free up mental space to stay connected to your body, says Anna Lutz, a registered dietitian in Raleigh, North Carolina. Mindful eating—listening without judgment to your body's hunger, fullness, and satisfaction signals—is an important part of the intuitive eating approach. Consider, "Did that last bite of steak taste as good as the first, or am I getting full?" "Would I find this broccoli more satisfying with a little salt or butter, or am I choking it down to check veggies off my list?"

Eat joyfully

Eating is meant to feel good. Food is comforting, it's communal, and it's delicious. "Taking unapologetic joy in food, especially in the foods we've been socialized to think are bad, is absolutely counter-cultural, radical—and really freaking fun," says Sole-Smith. When we freely allow ourselves to eat certain foods, they become more satiating than when we sneak them in during the trip home from work. Eating shouldn't just be about filling our bellies. Ideally, we should be able to say, "*Mmm*, I'm satisfied!"

TRY THIS: First give yourself permission to enjoy a variety of foods without guilt. Let this be your mantra: "There are no good or bad foods. I can eat whatever I want. If I listen to my body's signals, I will eat the right foods for me." When you have a couple of bites of pie and realize there will always be more pie, you don't feel the need to eat until you're stuffed. "One of the most beautiful things I see with people who go through the intuitive eating process is that they don't crave the thing they once binged on, because now it's always allowed," says Stefani Reinold, MD, MPH, a psychiatrist and the host of the podcast *It's Not About the Food.*

Second, make meals sensory events. Practice eating with a chef's mindset, suggests Murray. "Chefs would be devastated if they spent hours preparing a meal and knew that as you sat down to eat it, you overanalyzed every single calorie and milligram of salt or just scarfed it down—didn't even savor it," she says. "Sit down, taste it, and enjoy it."

Consider adding treats for your other senses: Set out flowers and put on relaxing music, says Scritchfield. Not every meal has to be candlelit, of course. A pit stop for a mediocre burger and fries is just one meal of thousands you'll eat in your lifetime, so you don't have to feel bad about it. Mindful, enjoyable eating is a goal, not a guilt trap.

Take a gentle approach to nutrition

With intuitive eating, nutrition is important, but don't think of it as a scolding taskmaster—merely a guide to what will keep your body feeling good. As you grow accustomed to intuitive eating, you can decide whether it's time for carrots...or carrot cake, says Scritchfield. During a relaxing dinner out with her daughters, she explains, she might savor that piece of cake. But between client appointments during the workday, she might choose energy-boosting carrots and hummus. The key: While there is a nutritional difference to these carrot foods, there is not a moral difference.

TRY THIS: To boost nutrition, think about what foods you can add rather than subtract, advises Murray. Increasing your intake of water, fruit, and vegetables is good for your health and doesn't require banning anything. And feel free to prepare vegetables however you like—yes, even with butter or olive oil or some ranch dressing. Nutrient-packed foods should satisfy the palate too.

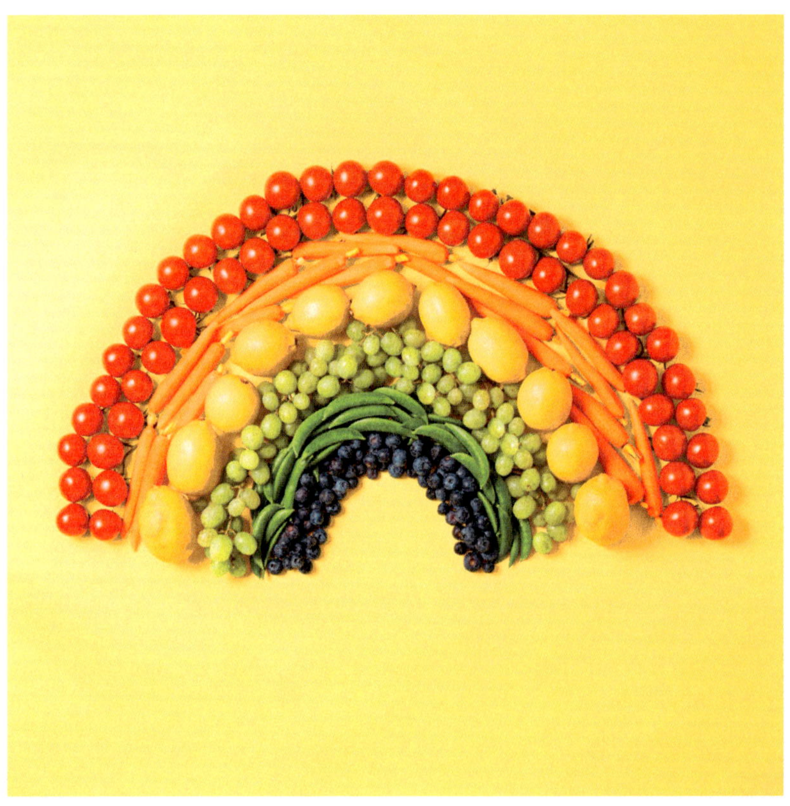

Be patient with yourself

Don't expect to drop all your food and weight baggage right away; the timing is different for everyone who explores intuitive eating. Many people worry that without lots of rules around eating, they'll immediately start gaining weight. And you might, if you were seriously restrictive before, says Reinold—but you may actually lose weight if you habitually kept eating after you were already full. Either way, it's OK: Weight naturally fluctuates, and pregnancies, age, and menopause will affect your body as well. "Acknowledging that can be uncomfortable at first," says Reinold. "But the result is freedom."

TRY THIS: To take the power (or panic) out of weight fluctuations, stop weighing yourself. Focus on more meaningful measures of health. For example, do you feel more energetic? Are you having fewer uncontrollable cravings? "I encourage people to try intuitive eating for three months just to get acquainted with it," says Murray. "It can definitely take a year to feel truly comfortable practicing it. It is very hard to move from the dieting mindset to the intuitive eating mindset." Be kind to yourself, no matter how long it takes. As Scritchfield puts it, "How much time do you think you're worth?"

THE SKEPTIC'S GUIDE TO INTUITIVE EATING

Will intuitive eating really help me think about food less? It sounds like I'll be thinking about food more.

It may seem like that, but eating intuitively means devoting more thought to your body and less to food. You move away from external cues (weight, looks, dietary restrictions) and toward internal cues (hunger, fullness, satisfaction, energy), going from an attitude of restriction to one of compassion for your body.

I'm supposed to eat only when I'm hungry, but how do I do that with a job and kids?

Rational thought is part of intuitive eating. If you're hungry at 5 and dinner isn't until 7, you could have a snack to take the edge off or just eat dinner earlier. The choice depends on your thoughts and values. Similarly, if you know you'll be starving after a two-hour midday work meeting, have a bigger breakfast or eat lunch earlier to avoid becoming ravenous.

Is intuitive eating meant for kids too?

Intuitive eating dietitians often suggest parents be responsible for the "what," "when," and "where" of eating (for example, when it's time to eat dinner and what is served). Kids can be responsible for the "which" and "how much" (which part of their lunch to eat first, how much to leave on their plates). ●

REAL SIMPLE

Vice President, Editor in Chief Liz Vaccariello
Creative Director Emily Kehe
Executive Editor Rory Evans
Executive Managing Editor Lavinel Savu
Photo Director Muzam Agha
Deputy Photo Editor Lawrence J. Whritenour Jr.

Mental Well-Being

Editorial Director Kostya Kennedy
Creative Director Gary Stewart
Editor Lisa Lombardi
Designer Ronnie Brandwein-Keats
Assistant Photo Editor Steph Durante
Writers Juli Fraga, Leslie Goldman, Ginny Graves, Sharon Holbrook, Marjorie Ingall, Hallie Levine, Sara Gaynes Levy, Jennifer King Lindley, Lisa Lombardi, Melanie Mannarino, Andrea Petersen, Holly Robinson, Laura Schocker, Maggie Seaver, Cassie Shortsleeve, Janet Siroto, Virginia Sole-Smith, Kimberly Truong
Copy Editor Ben Ake
Researcher Gillian Aldrich
Production Designer Sandra Jurevics
Premedia Trafficking Supervisor Tony Jungweber
Color Quality Analyst Pamela Powers

MEREDITH PREMIUM PUBLISHING
Vice President & Group Publisher Scott Mortimer
Vice President, Group Editorial Director Stephen Orr
Vice President, Marketing Jeremy Biloon
Director, Brand Marketing Jean Kennedy
Associate Director, Brand Marketing Bryan Christian
Senior Brand Manager Katherine Barnet

Editorial Director Kostya Kennedy
Creative Director Gary Stewart
Director of Photography Christina Lieberman
Editorial Operations Director Jamie Roth Major
Manager, Editorial Operations Gina Scauzillo

Special thanks Brad Beatson, Samantha Lebofsky, Kate Roncinske, Joel Van Liew, Laura Villano

MEREDITH NATIONAL MEDIA GROUP
President, Meredith Magazines Doug Olson
President, Consumer Products Tom Witschi
President, Chief Digital Officer Catherine Levene
Chief Marketing & Data Officer Alysia Borsa
Chief Revenue Officer Michael Brownstein
Marketing & Integrated Communications Nancy Weber

SENIOR VICE PRESIDENTS
Consumer Revenue Andy Wilson
Corporate Sales Brian Kightlinger
Research Solutions Britta Cleveland
Strategic Sourcing, Newsstand, Production Chuck Howell
Digital Sales Marla Newman
The Foundry Matt Petersen
Product & Technology Justin Law

VICE PRESIDENTS
Finance Chris Susil
Business Planning & Analysis Rob Silverstone
Consumer Marketing Steve Crowe
Brand Licensing Toye Cody, Sondra Newkirk
Corporate Communications Jill Davison
Vice President, Group Editorial Director Stephen Orr
Director, Editorial Operations & Finance Greg Kayko

MEREDITH CORPORATION
President & Chief Executive Officer Tom Harty
Chief Financial Officer Jason Frierott
Chief Development Officer John Zieser
Chief Strategy Officer Daphne Kwon
President, Meredith Local Media Group Patrick McCreery
Senior Vice President, Human Resources Dina Nathanson

Chairman Stephen M. Lacy
Vice Chairman Mell Meredith Frazier

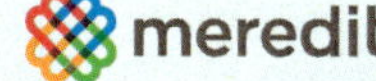

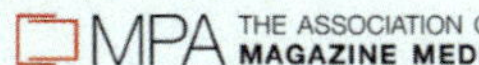

Published by Meredith Corporation
225 Liberty Street • New York, NY 10281

Printed in the U.S.A.

Photo and Illustration Credits

FRONT COVER
Martí Sans/Stocksy

BACK COVER
(Clockwise from top) Marc Tran/Stocksy; Trinette Reed/Stocksy; merla/Adobe Stock

TITLE PAGE
Baramee/Adobe Stock

CONTENTS
PP. 2–3 (from left) fortyforks/Adobe Stock; Westend61/Getty Images; Lloyd Dobbie/Blend Images LLC/Jacobs Stock Photography Ltd./Digital Vision/Getty Images; Caitlin Bensel

INTRODUCTION
P. 5 Ponomariova_Maria/iStock/Getty Images

CHAPTER ONE
PP. 6–7 kite_rin/Adobe Stock **PP. 8–9** Marina Suslova/Shutterstock **P. 11** 130920/Moment/Getty Images **P. 12** Trinette Reed/Stocksy **PP. 14–17** Klaus Vedfelt/Digital Vision/Getty Images (2) **PP. 18–22** Domenic Bahmann (3) **PP. 24–25** Westend61/Getty Images **P. 26** naka/Adobe Stock **P. 28** Lightfield Studios/Adobe Stock **PP. 30–31** AlisaRut/iStock/Getty Images **P. 32** Sky_melody/iStock/Getty Images

CHAPTER TWO
PP. 34–35 Hugh Taylor/Gallery Stock **PP. 36–37** New Africa/Adobe Stock **P. 39** Prostock-studio/Shutterstock **P. 40** Blaine Moats **PP. 42–43** karandaev/iStock/Getty Images **P. 44** Lloyd Dobbie/Blend Images LLC/Jacobs Stock Photography Ltd./Digital Vision/Getty Images **P. 45** Willie B. Thomas/Hinterhaus Productions/Digital Vision/Getty Images **P. 46** Wilaipon Pasawat/EyeEm/Getty Images **P. 47** Soubrette/iStock/Getty Images **PP. 48–49** Jörg Stöber/iStock/Getty Images **PP. 50–51** Photocreo Bednarek/Adobe Stock **P. 53** Yasu & Junko/Trunk Archive **PP. 54–57** Shout (3) **P. 58** Africa Studio/Adobe Stock **P. 60** Bonninstudio/Stocksy **PP. 62–66** Gracia Lam (3) **P. 67** Lea Csontos/Stocksy **PP. 68–73** Holly Andres (3)

CHAPTER THREE
PP. 74–75 Sara Forrest/Gallery Stock **PP. 76–79** Caitlin Bensel (2) **P. 80** mythja/Shutterstock **P. 83** Ali Harper/Stocksy **PP. 84–85** Maridav/Adobe Stock **P. 87** 9dream studio/Shutterstock **P. 88** Micky Wiswedel/Stocksy **P. 89** alexlesko/iStock/Getty Images **PP. 90–94** Peter Ardito (3) **P. 95** Ewa Ahlin/Johner RF/Getty Images **P. 96** Erickson Productions, Inc./Cavan Images

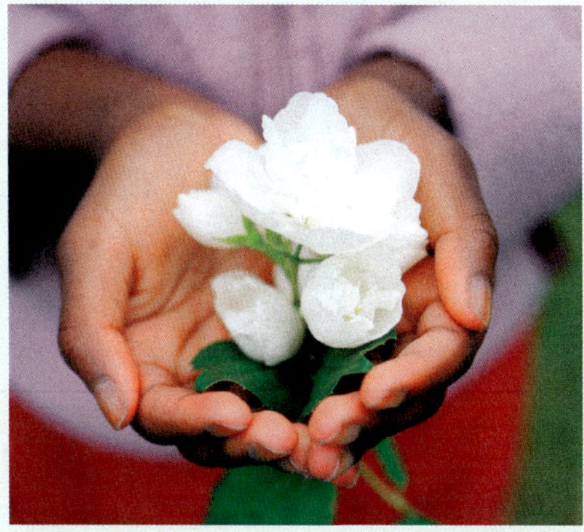

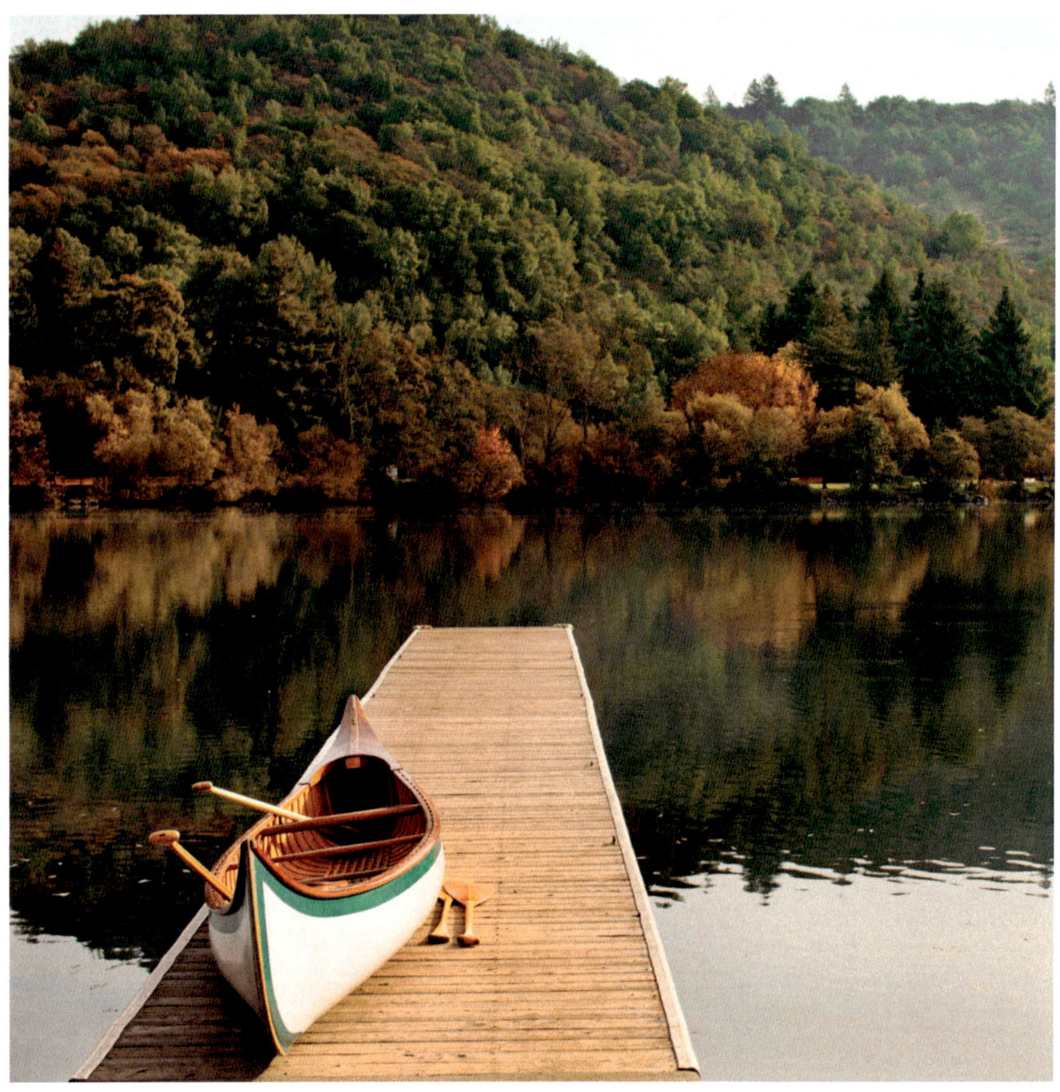

Fresh Air and Happiness

It isn't your imagination: Nature is healing. Getting out into the great outdoors—whether you're going on a summer beach stroll or a brisk winter hike—boosts the parasympathetic nervous system, decreasing stress and flooding the brain with feelings of calm. Indeed, a 2019 study found that folks who spend at least two hours a week in nature are more likely to rate their well-being as high compared with those who report no nature exposure.

Sara C. Mednick, PhD, the director of the University of California, Irvine, Sleep and Cognition Lab, chalks it up to how nature makes us feel connected to something bigger than ourselves. "The landscape changes in a natural cycle with the seasons, and you feel a sense of awe from the enormity of the big and small living things flourishing in the ecosystem," she says. "These emotions may have a system-wide anti-inflammatory effect, which can protect against depression."

Exercising outside? Even better. In a study led by Austrian sport scientists, adults who hiked outdoors for 45 minutes reported feeling happier, calmer, and more energized than those who walked for the same amount of time on an indoor treadmill. Urban dwellers can benefit too: Parks and gardens count as green spaces. —*Leslie Goldman*

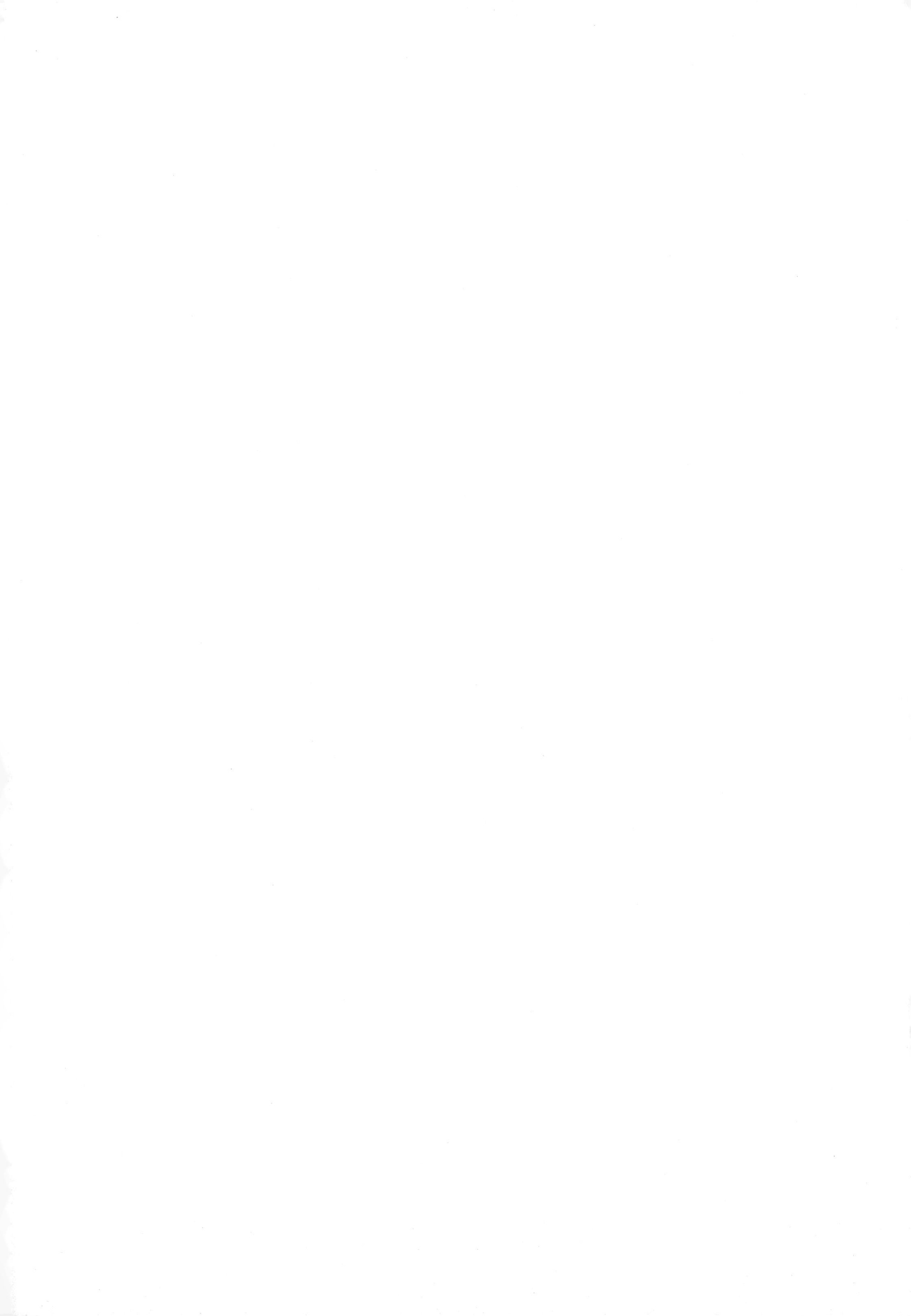

Made in the USA
Coppell, TX
21 May 2023

17089849R00059